Applying Quality Methodologies
to Improve Healthcare

Six Sigma, Lean Thinking, Balanced Scorecard, and More

Dawn Vonderheide-Liem, RN, MSN, CPHQ
Bud Pate, REHS

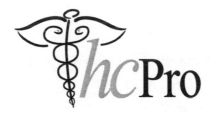

Dawn Vonderheide-Liem, RN, MSN, CPHQ, Co-author

Bud Pate, REHS, Co-author

Amy Anthony, Managing Editor

Matthew Cann, Group Publisher

Mike Mirabello, Senior Graphic Artist

Mike Michaud, Layout Artist

Jean St. Pierre, Creative Director

Shane Katz, Cover Designer

Arrangements can be made for quantity discounts. For more information, contact:

HCPro, Inc.
P.O. Box 1168
Marblehead, MA 01945
Telephone: 800/650-6787 or 781/639-1872
Fax: 781/639-2982
E-mail: *customerservice@hcpro.com*

Visit HCPro at its World Wide Web sites: *www.hcpro.com*, *www.hcmarketplace.com*

10/2004
20831

CONTENTS

Contents

Chapter Six: Balanced Scorecard .... .85

Chapter Seven: ISO 9000 .... .101

Chapter Eight: The Malcolm Baldrige National Quality Award .... .111

Chapter Nine: Rapid Cycle Testing .... .121

Contents

ABOUT THE AUTHORS

Dawn Vonderheide-Liem, RN, MSN, CPHQ

Dawn Vonderheide-Liem, RN, MSN, CPHQ, has been practicing performance improvement with Kaiser Permanente since 1990. Having earned her BSN and MSN at California State University, Los Angeles, she was a staff nurse at Kaiser during the 1970s and 1980s. She is responsible for performance improvement, patient safety, risk management, and infection control in an integrated system for both the Kaiser hospital and for the Southern California Permanente Medical Group in the Baldwin Park area. This system provides care for more than 220,000 members. Dawn has been awarded the Kaiser Permanente Leadership Award in 1998, 2000, 2001, and 2002.

She facilitates teams for business plan strategic goal deployment, root cause analysis, failure mode effects analysis, and medical center teams addressing both strategic and operational goals. She teaches performance improvement tools—most notably, statistical process control for healthcare—was one of the designers of training materials for failure mode and effect analysis for Southern California Kaiser Permanente.

She is a co-designer of the deployment methodology for addressing strategic goals for the medical center, which includes a medical center–level scorecard, the department-level scorecard and sharing successes through performance improvement storyboards.

Currently, she works at the Kaiser Permanente facility at Baldwin Park, California. She participated in the opening of that facility in 1998.

Bud Pate, REHS

Bud Pate, REHS, joined The Greeley Company after 15 years at Kaiser Permanente. Bud was responsible for a wide range of region-wide quality and compliance initiatives during his tenure at Kaiser in Southern California. He was responsible for standards and survey processes established by the Joint Commission on Accreditation of Healthcare Organizations (JCAHO), the Centers for Medicare & Medicaid Services, the California Department of Health Services (DHS), and the Office of Statewide Health Planning and Development. He also held leadership roles in Kaiser teams that developed industry-leading processes for the integration of health plan and hospital credentialing, moderate and deep sedation, and best practice–driven assessments of emergency departments (ED).

Before joining Kaiser Permanente in 1988, Bud was the supervisor of the Acute and Ancillary Services Section of the Los Angeles County Department of Health Services, Health Facilities Division. In that role, he was responsible for state licensing and Medicare/Medicaid certification activities for more than 150 general acute care hospitals, 200 home health agencies, and several dialysis and surgery clinics. Bud taught epidemiology and Washington Technical Institute in Washington, DC, prior to joining the LA County DHS.

A nationally recognized expert in healthcare operations and compliance, Bud chaired the Joint Committee on Accreditation of the California Healthcare Association and regional healthcare councils for many years. Bud represented the American Hospital Association on the JCAHO's Standards Review Task Force, the Hospital Advisory Committee, and other JCAHO work groups and panels that were part of the *Shared Visions–New Pathways*™ development effort.

Bud is a prolific and engaging speaker on a variety of topics, ranging from the JCAHO's survey process, mitigating ED overcrowding by improving patient flow, root cause analysis, the federal Emergency Medical Treatment and Active Labor Act, and other compliance and quality topics. He has lectured in many settings, including programs sponsored by the National Institute for Occupational Safety, the Institute for Healthcare Improvement (IHI), the University of California at Los Angeles, California, State University in Northridge, and the California Medical Association. He has authored articles on accreditation and root cause analysis, including an article published by IHI on the diagnosis and treatment of blame. His latest effort (with Derenda Pete of InSight Advantage) is *Solving Emergency Department Overcrowding: Successful Approaches to a Chronic Problem*, a book that was published in 2003 by HCPro, Inc.

Bud received his Bachelor of Arts degree from the University of California at Los Angeles and a Certificate in Environmental Management from the University of Southern California, School of Public Administration. He is a registered environmental health specialist in California.

PREFACE

This book will help quality professionals and hospital leaders navigate the litany of terms like Six Sigma, Lean Thinking, Balanced Scorecards, ISO, and Baldrige to design a program that will be effective in their organization. The book is a reference for answering frequently asked questions, like the following:

Question: Does the Joint Commission on Accreditation of Healthcare Organizations (JCAHO) require a hospital to use Six Sigma or Lean Thinking?

Answer: No. However, JCAHO and the external realities that drive healthcare in the third millennium demand improvement, no matter how it is accomplished. We are challenged to enhance patient safety, unclog patient flow, maximize financial performance, increase patient satisfaction, better serve our communities, and ensure employee commitment. Six Sigma, Lean Thinking and the other approaches discussed in this book have a proven track record of success in other industries, and healthcare continues to experiment, as it has for the last two decades, to find the right fit.

Question: Is Six Sigma or Lean Thinking really different?

Answer: Yes and no.
Yes, there are some new approaches to improvement embedded in Six Sigma and other methods described in this book.

No, the fundamental principles are the same as those first described in Walter Shewhart's seminal 1931 text, *Economic Control of Quality of Manufactured Product*.

Question: Do Six Sigma and Lean Thinking work for healthcare?

Answer: Sometimes.

These approaches have been found very effective in a number of other industries. However, they have not been used long enough nor widely enough to declare either a clear "winner" in the race to be the method of choice for healthcare improvement.

Question: What is the right approach for my institution?

Answer: Sorry, you'll have to read the entire book to answer this one.

Through these pages, we will distinguish Six Sigma, Lean Thinking, TQM, and other quality improvement approaches from one another. We will also discuss the true key to successful improvement: effective leadership.

This book will not make you an expert in any particular improvement technique. This book will, however, give you enough information to decide whether a change in your approach to improvement is indicated. It will also help you focus on one or two candidate models should you decide that a change is necessary.

INTRODUCTION

QUALITY IMPROVEMENT AND
THE HEALTHCARE ENVIRONMENT

JCAHO: From prescribed methods to expected outcomes

We've been around quality for long enough to remember when the Joint Commission on Accreditation of Healthcare Organizations (JCAHO) required chart audits as the approach to quality. Starting with Dr. Ernest Codman's categorization of surgical outcomes at the turn of the 20th century, the American College of Surgeons and its successor, the JCAHO, have required attention to quality as a core requirement for accreditation.

In recent times, JCAHO has moved away from requiring specific monitors, such as drug use evaluation or surgical case review. Instead, the JCAHO has adopted a multi-phased approach to improving quality in the hopes of finally making a demonstrable impact on quality.

- After a number of fits and starts, JCAHO has finally settled on a core of clinical indicators that all hospitals will measure.

- These measures then feed into an overall structure of data definition, collection, and analysis that is expected to lead to improvements.

Exactly how to make these improvements is left to the institution.

Learning from other industries

Other industries, like manufacturing, retail, service, and manufacturing have long lived in a sink-or-swim world. The marketplace determines which ventures succeed and which disappear. Just ask anyone with frequent-flier miles on Pan American or stockholders in Montgomery Ward; to these industries, quality is satisfaction and satisfaction is survival.

Hospitals and other healthcare institutions have been insulated from this world in many ways, especially since the advent of Medicare. But times are changing. Hospitals across the country are closing and consolidating. Escalating costs have led to real competition in the marketplace.

It is not surprising, then, that healthcare leaders are turning more than ever to other industries for lessons in quality and survival.

About quality methods

Virtually any quality method, if properly applied, will work. And any quality method is also subject to failure. So, which method is best for YOUR organization?

Total Quality Management (TQM) came to healthcare in the late 1980s. It seemed to be the answer to our problems:

- It was working well in other industries.
- It seemed simple enough, at least to a system engineer.
- It appeared to be a comfortable fit for healthcare.

Why, then, did TQM lose favor? Why is it now passé?

Six Sigma, Lean Thinking, International Standards Organization (ISO), and Baldrige are among the current contenders for improvement method of choice. Will any of them emerge as THE best path to positive and lasting change? Or will their glow fade to be replaced by the next "flavor of the month"?

Choosing a quality approach

Why so many different approaches? Are some better than others? If one is best, why are the others also popular? Why has one method not grown to dominate the field?

Quality methods are, in fact, management tools. They are ways of leading an endeavor and, therefore, their success has as much to do with the style of the leaders as it does with the objective effectiveness of the system.

Critical mass

Adopting a new quality system is costly. It involves change, which is never easy. Like all high-profile change efforts, they are not without risk. There is

- the cost of training
- the cost of lost momentum
- the risk of a high-profile failure

It is not surprising, therefore, that changing to a new quality approach is not undertaken lightly. There must be critical mass. In our experience, leaders change systems for one or more of the following reasons:

- The previous quality system failed to produce meaningful momentum for positive change.
- The institution is under significant pressure to improve: it's facing declining marketshare or profit margin or is scrambling to avoid or recover from a crisis.
- Executive leadership is new and needs to provide a new roadmap to the future, avoiding drift.

So many choices

Consultants are always ready to lead you toward a brighter tomorrow through the adoption of their system. There is no shortage of quality approaches, each with countless variations. Each product and each variation has its own success story.

Six Sigma is very popular at the moment. At its core, Six Sigma promises a measurable return to the financial bottom line with each project selected. Six Sigma applications are very structured and require a return on investment for each project undertaken. Most projects are linked to the strategic goals of the organization, virtually guaranteeing the focus and support of senior leadership. Yet even with such a heavy focus on the bottom line, Six Sigma implementations often fail—by some estimates, as often as 20% of the time.

You may be considering Toyota's **Lean Thinking** methods. Like Six Sigma, Lean Thinking projects focus on important "pain points" in organizational performance. Lean Thinking is dedicated to elimination of waste—creating a return to the bottom line through improved efficiency. But there are many failed Lean Thinking implementations as well.

Balanced Scorecards seem like a good way to understand organizational performance, thereby keeping the institution on track and improving. But understanding one's performance and doing something about it are two very different issues. Monitoring performance without support for improvement doesn't work—at least in the long run. Therefore, Balanced Scorecards must be combined with another overall quality improvement structure in order to be effective.

Standard-based improvement approaches, such as **ISO 9000,** the **Malcolm Baldrige National Quality Award** and **JCAHO's performance improvement** expectations, provide frameworks for improvement without providing the specific methods to achieve it. Such frameworks are quite useful, but incomplete.

Benchmarking and **quality circles** are older approaches that are still used to good effect by some institutions within the framework of **TQM** or **continuous quality improvement.**

Learn from history

Before you decide on a new method, take a critical look at what didn't work in the past:

- Was the prior improvement method deficient (unlikely), or was it poorly implemented (usually)?

- Were there absolutely no successes with the old method (unlikely), or were the successes too few or minor/marginal issues (usually)?

- Was leadership patient with the old system, allowing it the time and attention to work (unlikely), or were they disappointed when the improvements were not quick enough (usually)?

- Was the old system aimed at the truly important issues with significance for the future of the institution (unlikely), or was it aimed at the small issues such as report turnaround times or crash chart readiness (usually)?

The factor that leads to success or failure is often the least tangible one: the culture of the organization. In the end, the effective improvement method will be the one that best fits the culture. That is, choose the method the organization will really use.

Just as in our personal lives there is no one diet and no one exercise regimen that is "the best." When trying to lose weight, some people do well on Weight Watchers, others prefer South Beach or Atkins, some opt for surgery, and some can't lose weight no matter what they do. Creating good habits and sticking to a system for the long term is what works best of all.

Therefore, ask yourself, "Is this institution most likely to sustain Six Sigma or Lean Thinking?" Do we have a stable leadership champion who will embrace TQM? Is our corporate structure suited to a standards-based approach, such as ISO 9000? Answers to questions like these will lead you to the right improvement method.

CHAPTER ONE

TOTAL QUALITY MANAGEMENT

CHAPTER ONE

TOTAL QUALITY MANAGEMENT

ELEVATOR DESCRIPTION OF TOTAL QUALITY MANAGEMENT

Quick: You have a two-floor ride in an elevator with your CEO and medical director, and they want to know about Total Quality Management (TQM).

TQM is a structured system of continuous improvement with employee involvement and training, problem-solving teams, statistical methods, identification and elimination of waste in the production of products or delivery of services, and recognition that the system, not the people using it, produces inefficiencies.

In 1931, **Walter A. Shewhart,** a statistician at the Hawthorne plant at Western Electric, began to develop modern statistical process control: that is the measurement of processes over time to study the pattern of variation. At the same time, he provided the basis for the philosophy of continuous process improvement.

> Total = Involving everyone and all processes
>
> Quality = Meeting customer requirements
>
> Management = The way we do business

It was Shewhart who developed the never-ending approach to process improvement we've come to know as "plan-do-check-act," or the "Shewhart cycle."

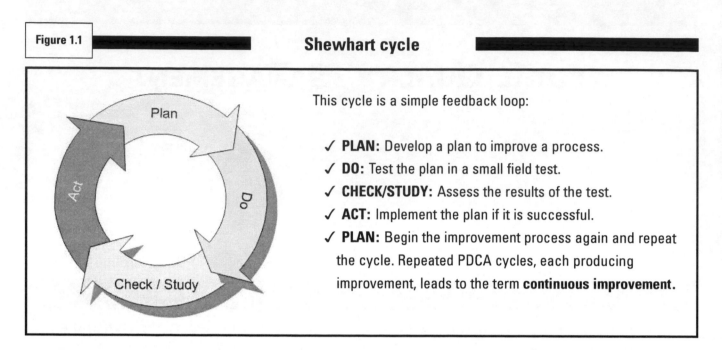

Figure 1.1   **Shewhart cycle**

This cycle is a simple feedback loop:

✓ **PLAN:** Develop a plan to improve a process.
✓ **DO:** Test the plan in a small field test.
✓ **CHECK/STUDY:** Assess the results of the test.
✓ **ACT:** Implement the plan if it is successful.
✓ **PLAN:** Begin the improvement process again and repeat the cycle. Repeated PDCA cycles, each producing improvement, leads to the term **continuous improvement.**

After World War II, Shewhart and **W. Edwards Deming** presented lectures to American engineers and managers involved in manufacturing about statistical process control (SPC) and the wartime refinements to it. Many engineers who attended these lectures were convinced, and they adopted the SPC philosophy. However, as the demand for products increased after the war, most companies were more interested in meeting quotas than in a quality of the product or its fitness for use.

In the 1950s, the Japanese asked Shewhart, Deming, and a third American statistician, **Joseph Juran,** to help them improve their war-torn economy. By implementing the principles of TQM, Japan experienced dramatic economic growth. American industry, however, showed little interest in the technique. Over time, products from Japan became better and cheaper and became the products of choice over those produced in America.

Then, in 1982, Deming published his book *Out of the Crisis*, which laid out his approach (Deming's "14 Points") to statistical process control and improvement theory. Having witnessed the success of such philosophies in Japan, now a major competitor for U.S. markets, many American companies adopted the 14 Points as the centerpiece of their quality philosophies.

Juran and **Philip B. Crosby** developed a slightly different approach to continuous improvement. Nevertheless, their philosophies were very similar to Deming's methods.

Today, most organizations that have successfully internalized a philosophy of continuous improvement have followed the approach of Shewhart, Deming, Juran, or Crosby. These organizations include manufacturing, service, health, education, military, and government agencies.

| Figure 1.2 | **Pioneers of total quality management** |

Shewhart	Statistical Process Control Plan, Do, Check, Act Cycle
Deming	14 Points for Total Quality Management Common causes of variation
Juran	Quality is fitness for use The quality trilogy: quality planning, quality improvement, and quality control
Crosby	Quality is free Zero defects

DEMING'S 14 STEPS

Based on his work with Japanese managers and others, Deming outlined 14 steps that managers in any type of organization can take to implement a TQM program.

1. Create constancy of purpose for improvement of product and service. Constancy of purpose requires innovation, investment in research and education, continuous improvement of product and service, maintenance of equipment, furniture and fixtures, and new aids to production.

2. Adopt the new philosophy. Management must undergo a transformation and begin to believe in quality products and services.

3. Cease dependence on mass inspection. Inspect products and services only enough to identify ways to improve the process.

4. End the practice of awarding business on price tag alone. The lowest-priced goods are not always the highest quality; choose a supplier based on its record of improvement and then make a long-term commitment to it.

5. Improve constantly and forever the system of product and service. Improvement is not a one-time effort; management is responsible for leading the organization into the practice of continual improvement in quality and productivity.

6. Institute training and retraining. Workers need to know how to do their jobs correctly, even if that means learning new skills.

DEMING'S 14 STEPS (CONT.)

7. Institute leadership. Managers must discover and remove the barriers that prevent staff from taking pride in what they do.

8. Drive out fear. People often fear reprisal if they "make waves" at work. Managers need to create an environment where workers can express concerns with confidence.

9. Break down barriers between staff areas. Managers should promote teamwork by helping staff in different areas/departments work together. Fostering interrelationships among departments encourages higher quality decision-making.

10. Eliminate slogans, exhortations, and targets for the workforce. Using slogans alone, without investigation into the processes of the workplace, can be offensive to workers because they imply that a better job could be done. Managers need to learn real ways of motivating people in their organizations.

11. Eliminate numerical quotas. Quotas impede quality more than any other working condition: They leave no room for improvement. Workers need to have the flexibility to give customers the level of service they need.

12. Remove barriers to pride of workmanship. Give workers respect and feedback about how they are doing their jobs.

13. Institute a vigorous program of education and retraining. With continuous improvement, job descriptions will change. As a result, employees will need to be educated and retrained so they will be successful at new job responsibilities.

14. Take action to accomplish the transformation. Management must work as a team to carry out the previous 13 steps.

The key to TQM

TQM is mainly concerned with continuous improvement in all work, from high-level strategic planning and decision-making to detailed application of work elements wherever they may be performed. TQM believes that mistakes can be avoided and defects can be prevented. With that belief, it leads to continuously improving results in all aspects of work processes, including people, technology, and machine capabilities.

✓ The key to improving the quality of a product is improving the component processes that define, produce, and support it.

✓ The customer at the end of the production system is part of the production process and must become involved in its improvement.

✓ Process problems must be eliminated or radically reduced.

✓ Managers must provide training and tools, measure the process, review the process, and improve performance with the help of those who are part of the process.

GOALS OF TQM

✓ Standardize repetitive work

✓ Describe goals of the process, thus providing an objective way to determine whether a particular result meets the client needs and expectations

✓ Agree about how to measure the process to determine the variability and the expected tolerances, if any, of the expected results

✓ Set measures, including SPC whenever possible, so you can identify quickly sources of deviations between expected results and actual results

✓ Create a step-by-step plan of action for problem solving to find the root cause of problems and to identify action plans to prevent further repetition of such problems, which normally result in changing procedures or in training employees to reinforce existing procedures

✓ Use ongoing measures to check the success of the action plans and determine whether there needs to be additional action

A central principle of TQM is that although people make mistakes, most of them are caused—or at least permitted—by faulty systems and processes.

✓ Anyone can make a mistake, from the best, most experienced employee to the newest and least experienced hire.

✓ Mistakes primarily result from defective systems rather than defective people.

✓ Therefore, the root causes of mistakes can be identified and eliminated/reduced by changing the process.

There are three important approaches to reducing mistakes:

1. **Preventing** them (i.e., mistake-proofing or Poka-Yoke).
2. **Detecting** them early to prevent them from being passed to the next operation in the process.
3. **Stopping production** until the process can be corrected.

Measuring processes and process variability

To manage quality, you must use objective measures of performance to understand how well the process is working. But no system and no process is constant—All systems produce variable results.

This concept of process variability forms the heart of statistical process control (SPC). For example, the amount of time it takes you to drive from home to work is different every day. Some days your drive is 33 minutes, some days it takes 30 minutes and, some days it takes 36 minutes. Some days you encounter a slow driver, other days you stop to talk to a neighbor, and other days you make every green light (then stop to buy a lottery ticket). This type of variation is inherent to all systems—the drive to and from the office and cardiovascular surgery alike.

There are two types of variation within a process:

1. **Natural process variation,** frequently called **common cause** or **system variation,** is the natural fluctuations inherent to normal functioning of the process.
2. **Special cause variation** results from something that is not a normal part of the process.

The stop lights and the slow cars are part of the normal traffic pattern and account for a large part of the **common cause** variation in your drive to work. Having a flat tire on the way to work, however, would be a **special cause** of variation.

| Figure 1.3 | **Control charts of daily drive time** |

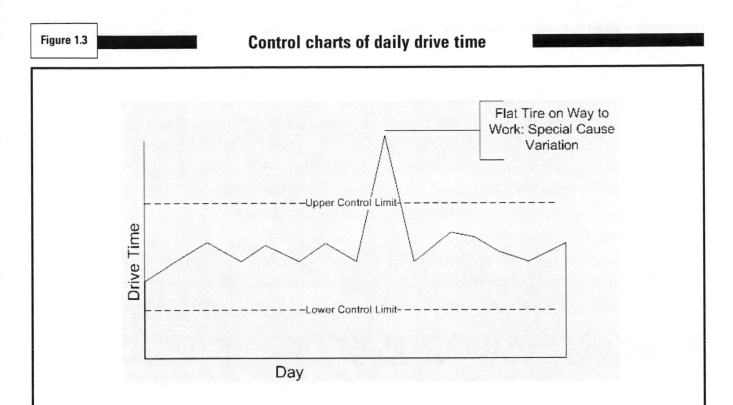

Flat Tire on Way to Work: Special Cause Variation

Upper Control Limit

Drive Time

Lower Control Limit

Day

A control chart is a run chart with upper and lower control limits. The above chart shows drive times to work. The drive time for most days varies only a little due to missed traffic lights and variations in traffic flow. However, one drive time is longer than normal (past the upper control limit) because the driver got a flat tire on the way to work. The routine fluctuations are "common cause" variations. The drive time for the day with the flat tire is a "special cause" variation: the cause was not part of the normal system.

Shewhart developed a system to help us distinguish between **common** and **special** cause variation. Today we call that system **SPC.**

SPC is a method of charting a process to determine quickly whether a process is "out of control" due to a special cause or whether the process is just undergoing natural variation due to common causes. Knowledge of basic SPC is fundamental to TQM.

TQM aims to reduce **both** common and special cause variation. Reduced variation makes the process more predictable and keeps process output closer to the desired value or outcome. The PDCA cycle, repeated many times, provides the mechanism for accomplishing continuing variation reduction or continuous improvement.

Teams—employee involvement and training

Because people closest to the work know the process best, they must be included in any improvement team. Such a team approach to the "PLAN" phase of the Shewhart cycle is key to TQM.

Facilitators or others trained in improvement methodologies may guide this team, which meet and review the overall process—usually using a flow diagram—and get data to understand how well the process is performing. However, the team should be put in place only when there is clear support for the improvement at the right level of the organization, with the corresponding commitment of resources (time, materials, training, and other support to make it work).

A word of caution: The team's work can be slow when the project is not clearly identified, when the need for improvement is not clear or is not supported whole heartedly by the sponsor, and when the team becomes unmanageable for the facilitator due to behaviors of the team members.

OBTAIN THE RIGHT LEVEL OF SPONSORSHIP

✓ If the process to improve involves a number of different departments, it should be sponsored by senior leadership.

✓ If the process to improve involves physicians, sponsorship should also include a medical staff committee.

✓ If the process to improve is contained entirely within one department, only the department manager needs to sponsor the team.

TQM tools

There are many improvement tools available; however the following basic improvement tools are commonly used due to their broad application. These tools are often very useful in identifying root-cause problems and guiding the success of new processes. Taken together, they form a powerful set of instruments to help the team work through the PDCA cycle.

> ✓ **Pareto diagram**—focuses on problems that offer the greatest potential for improvement
> ✓ **Control chart**—focuses on detecting and monitoring process variation over time
> ✓ **Run charts**—focuses on performance measure of a process for trends or patterns over a specific period of time
> ✓ **Flow charts**—identifies the actual flow or sequence of events in a process

---

✓ **Histograms**—demonstrates the frequency distribution of a process

✓ **Brainstorming**—collects ideas on a topic in a way that is free of criticism and judgment

✓ **Cause and effect diagram** (also known as the **Ishikawa diagram** or **fishbone diagram**)—identifies, explores, and displays in increasing detail all of the possible causes related to a problem to lead to discovery of its root cause

Implementation of TQM—Leadership required! (aka "How to avoid failure")

Implementing TQM requires the commitment, sponsorship, resources, encouragement, and focus of senior leadership. It cannot be led from outside the operational chain of command.

Conduct an assessment of the current state of the organization to make sure the need for change is clear and that TQM is an appropriate strategy. Leadership styles and organizational culture must be congruent with TQM. If they are not, work on them to avoid/delay TQM implementation until favorable conditions exist.

You may need to use outside consultants to have a robust application. Consultants can bring a wealth of knowledge regarding the TQM process and have the experience to know when there is a problem with implementation. Consultants also can bring suggestions for dealing with the problems encountered. Choose consultants based on their prior relevant experience and their commitment to adapting the process to fit organizational needs. Remember, however, that although consultants will be invaluable with initial training of staff and TQM system design, employees (management and others) should be actively involved in TQM implementation. After receiving training they can train other employees. Establish a collaborative relationship with consultants, clear role definitions, and specification of activities.

Implementing TQM will be a difficult, comprehensive, and long-term process. *Leaders who think this will be a quick fix to their problems will be disappointed.* They will declare the TQM *methodology* as a failure when, in fact, it was their implementation effort that failed. To avoid this problem, leaders will need to

- maintain their commitment
- keep the process visible
- provide the necessary support
- listen carefully to customers
- maximize employee involvement in design of the system
- hold people accountable for the results

Always keep in mind that TQM should be *purpose driven*. By being clear about the organization's vision for the future and staying focused on it leadership will find TQM to be a powerful technique for unleashing employee creativity and potential, reducing bureaucracy and costs, and improving customer service.

TQM RESOURCES

Arthur M. Schneiderman, "Are there Limits to TQM?" *Strategy & Business,* Issue 11, Second Quarter (1998).

Michael Brassard and Diane Ritter, "Walter Shewhart—The Grandfather of Total Quality Management Memory Jogger" *www.Skymark. com* (accessed October 2004).

W. E. Deming, *Out of the crisis.* (Cambridge, MA: Massachusetts Institute of Technology, Center for Advanced Engineering Study, 1986).

CHAPTER TWO

BENCHMARKING

BENCHMARKING

ELEVATOR DESCRIPTION OF BENCHMARKING

Quick: You have a two-floor ride in an elevator with your CEO and medical director and they want to know about benchmarking.

Benchmarking is identifying the highest standard of performance, understanding the process it takes to get that performance, and adapting and applying standard and process to improve your own performance.

The purpose of benchmarking is to understand what someone else is doing to produce a high level of performance and then using that knowledge to help improve your own level of performance. Many confuse benchmarking with collecting and using comparative data, but

✓ the use of reference or comparative data is very useful to judge your level of performance, however it is not, by itself, "benchmarking."

✓ identifying a "benchmark" involves finding the highest achievable level of performance for the specific processes being measured.

Benchmarking is usually done within an industry, but it can also be done between organizations in different industries that have similar processes. In fact, organizations sometimes achieve better results by benchmarking a process across industries. Doing so tends to stimulate the challenging of one's assumptions about the way a process must be done. For example, hospitals often benchmark customer service with "best practices" in the hotel industry, such as those of the Ritz Carlton.

Variations in benchmarking include the following:

✓ "Best practice" studies
✓ Cooperative benchmarking
✓ Competitive benchmarking

"Best practice" studies

These are studies and lists of what works best. Although useful for benchmarking research, they are not useful as measurements of performance because what works the best for an organization in its specific environment may not work the same way in another environment. Therefore, these studies can be useful stimulators, but they are not "benchmarks" per se.

Cooperative benchmarking

Cooperative benchmarking is done with the cooperation of the organization being studied, or the benchmark "partner." The entity chosen as the benchmark partner often is one that has "best practices" in the area of interest or that has won a major national or international quality award. Internal audit departments are increasingly interested in this method.

This process includes obtaining measures of key production functions within the overall process, not just of the overall performance level. In addition, the organization studies the differences between their process and the "benchmark" process.

Competitive benchmarking

Competitive benchmarking, as the name implies, is the study and measurement of a high-performing competitor's process without its cooperation. Competitive benchmarking tends to be less effective than cooperative benchmarking because it is more difficult to discover what produces the desired effect—you don't have the cooperation of the benchmark organization.

Benchmarking steps

There are many versions of benchmarking steps used by very successful organizations. AT&T has 12, Xerox uses 10, Alcoa has six, and others recommend seven or eight. The simplest framework is recommended by GOAL/QPC, which has six steps (keyed to the Shewhart cycle of continuous improvement):

1. **Plan** (plan)
2. **Research** (plan)
3. **Observe** (do)

4. **Analyze** (do)

5. **Adapt** (check)

6. **Improve** (act)

| Figure 2.1 | 6-step benchmarking process |

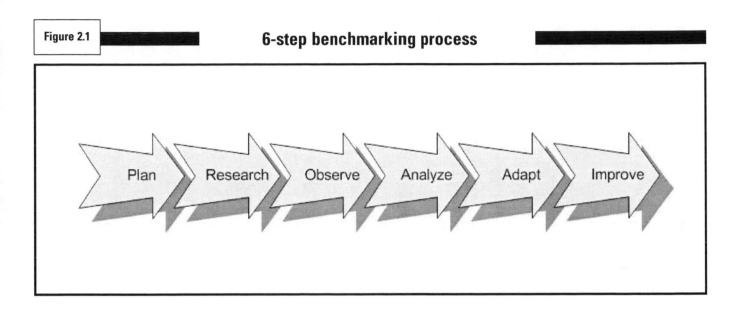

Benchmarking is a part of the TQM system, and it relates well to other TQM initiatives.

Benchmarking is not a one-time project. It is a continuous improvement strategy and a change-management process. Once the process begins, the entity should continue to benchmark against "best practices" in order to improve continuously.

BENCHMARKING REFERENCES

"Benchmarking for Healthcare." Benchmarking Strategies for Health Care Management *www.abhc.org/* (accessed October 2004).

H. James Harrington, *High Performance Benchmarking: 20 Steps to Success.*
Robert Damelio, *The Basics of Benchmarking.*

CHAPTER THREE

QUALITY CIRCLES

QUALITY CIRCLES

Quick: You have a two-floor ride in an elevator with your CEO and medical director and they want to know about quality circles.

A quality circle is a small group of six to 12 employees doing similar work who voluntarily meet regularly to identify improvements in their respective work areas using proven techniques for analyzing and solving work-related problems.

The concept of the quality circle recognizes the value of the worker as a human being, as someone who willingly participates, and as someone who brings to the job wisdom, intelligence, experience, attitudes and feelings.

The quality circle concept is a

- ✓ form of participation management
- ✓ human resource development technique
- ✓ problem-solving technique

A quality circle is most effective and efficient when you use the appropriate organizational structure, which depends on your industry and organization. Any structure, however, will follow the same basic framework, which consists of the following elements:

✓ The quality circle steering committee is headed by the leadership team. The committee establishes policy and plans and directs the program. It meets regularly—usually once a month—to provide oversight.

✓ Quality circle members are usually staff members and attend as many meetings as possible. They are the source of the new ideas and suggested approaches to solving problems and improving performance.

✓ The quality circle decides the frequency of its meetings.

✓ Quality circle members receive training on TQM problem-solving techniques and group dynamics.

✓ The quality circle leader is from management and is responsible for organizing the meetings and otherwise supporting the group.

✓ A quality circle facilitator is available to assist the quality circle leader and the team. The quality circle facilitator usually has multiple quality circles to assist.

✓ A quality circle coordinator provides coordination, supervises the work of the facilitators, and monitors the overall quality circle program.

✓ The quality circle uses basic problem solving techniques rooted in TQM, as such as brainstorming, Pareto diagrams, cause and effect diagrams, data collection, and data analysis. They may also use other basic tools such as tables, bar charts, histograms, line graphs, scatter grams, and control charts.

Steps in the quality circle process

Like other TQM techniques, the quality circle uses sequential steps to improve process. Although there is variation in the number and organization of the specific steps, the approach below is common to all circles and is keyed to the Shewhart cycle of continuous improvement:

1. Identify the problem (plan)
2. Select the problem (plan)
3. Analyze the problem (do)
4. Generate alternative solutions (do)
5. Select the most appropriate solution (do)
6. Prepare a plan of action (check)
7. Present solution to management for approval (check)
8. Implement approved solution (act)

Although quality circles are not commonly seen in the healthcare industry, aspects of the quality circle concept are used frequently. For example, unit-based teams or multiple disciplinary teams often are put together to solve problems within the work group or patient or service processes.

QUALITY CIRCLES RESOURCES

Quality Circles, Public Works Department, Government of Maharashtra. Go to *www.mahapwd.com/circulars/default.asp* for more information (accessed October 2004).

CHAPTER FOUR

SIX SIGMA

CHAPTER FOUR

SIX SIGMA

ELEVATOR DESCRIPTION OF SIX SIGMA

Quick: You have a two-floor ride in an elevator with your CEO and medical director and they want to know about Six Sigma.

Six Sigma is a highly structured and disciplined process to eliminate defects, waste, and quality problems. The resulting improved performance costs less and returns money to the bottom line.

Origins of the term 'Six Sigma'

It's impossible to go into the business section of your local book store without being accosted by dozens of titles proclaiming the virtues of Six Sigma. But when one looks at the tools and scans the table of contents, Six Sigma doesn't seem to be really that different from other improvement systems. Questions begin to arise:

- Why do people spend so much money becoming Black Belts and Green Belts?
- Why has Six Sigma taken off so dramatically?
- How do I decide whether it's right for my organization?

Six Sigma is an approach to quality that, in recent years, has been widely adopted in other industries and has yielded dramatic improvements in business performance by

- having a **precise understanding** of customer requirements
- **eliminating** defects from existing processes, products, or services

---

Sigma |σ| is a letter in the Greek alphabet that, by convention, is used to represent one standard deviation. Remember that bell-shaped curve from Psychology 101 or beginning statistics? In a perfect bell-shaped curve (Figure 4.1) that represents frequency of defects per opportunity, about 95% of the occurrences fall within two standard deviations (2σ) above or below the mean.

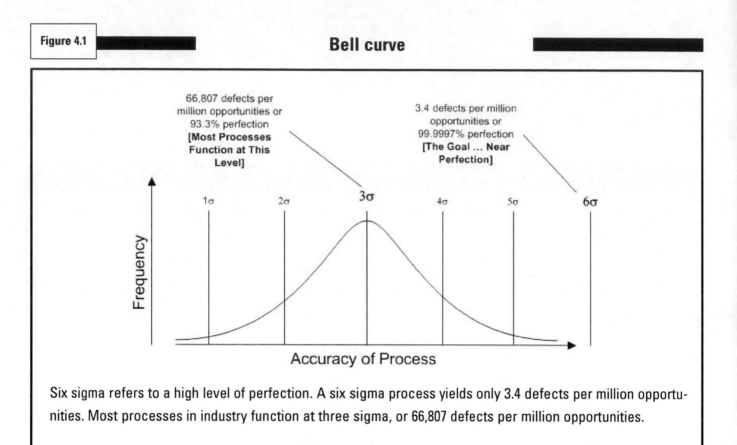

Figure 4.1   **Bell curve**

66,807 defects per million opportunities or 93.3% perfection
[Most Processes Function at This Level]

3.4 defects per million opportunities or 99.9997% perfection
[The Goal ... Near Perfection]

1σ   2σ   3σ   4σ   5σ   6σ

Frequency

Accuracy of Process

Six sigma refers to a high level of perfection. A six sigma process yields only 3.4 defects per million opportunities. Most processes in industry function at three sigma, or 66,807 defects per million opportunities.

Because this approach to quality aims to reduce defects, six sigma (6σ) refers to the number of defects that are six standard deviations below the mean. The ultimate goal is to perform so accurately relative to customers' specifications that there are only **3.4 defects per one million opportunities.**

This goal is laudable to be sure. Unfortunately, however, the goal of many organizations today is to operate at around two to three sigma. A performance of 2σ has a defect rate of about **308,000** per million opportunities. 3σ performance translates into **66,800** defects per million opportunities.

Imagine how much money an industry could save if it didn't have to do all that rework. Imagine how reliable its customers would perceive it to be. Isn't it far better to eliminate waste than to terminate employees when it comes time to trim costs?

Motorola and General Electric

The credit for the term "Six Sigma" and the quality process it represents goes to a Motorola engineer named Bill Smith. Motorola, which owns the Six Sigma trademark, was actually able to achieve performance at the 6σ (3.4 defects per million) level using Smith's approach. Improving performance to this level meant dramatic enhancements to Motorola's financial bottom line and is credited for keeping the company in business.

When Jack Welch was president of General Electric, he committed his company to a Six Sigma process and brought the method to further prominence. He realized that Six Sigma was more than a quality tool: It was entirely different approach to management. To make Six Sigma work Welch realized he would have to fund and increase training and dedicate his "best and brightest" to becoming "Black Belts" or projects leaders.

Motorola's and GE's investments paid off—big time. And now everyone is looking to Six Sigma as THE path to improvement.

So what makes Six Sigma different?

Many people think of Six Sigma as a quality control tool. But Six Sigma is a profound change in the leadership approach and culture of an organization, focusing on solutions to problems with the most return on the investment.

What are the hallmarks of a Six Sigma organization?

- **Structure:** Six Sigma is highly structured, with teams, committees, and a hierarchy of oversight and support structures.

- **Resources:** Six Sigma is not cheap. It demands the dedication of significant human resources and a willingness to engage outside experts to make the process work.

- **Customer focus:** Quality is rigorously defined in terms of the customer's specifications.

- **Error reduction:** Six Sigma approaches aim to reduce error and, thereby, contribute to the financial success of an organization.

- **Bottom line:** If, at the end of the day, the bottom line has not been enhanced, a Six Sigma project is a failure, regardless of the other wonderful fruits of the effort.

The idea, then, is to demand perfection.

Six Sigma incorporates the principles of Total Quality Management, and makes additions:

Black Belts: With imagery borrowed from martial arts, the Black Belt is a well-trained expert in process improvement and statistical analysis. When a Black Belt participates on a team, the expected return should be approximately $175,000 to $230,000 to the bottom line. Black Belts can typically complete four to five projects a year. Being a Black Belt is a full-time job.

Green Belts receive less training than Black Belts and continue in their regular work roles and responsibilities while supporting the Black Belt.

CORE SIX SIGMA PRINCIPLES

Improve performance by selecting projects that focus on

- customer satisfaction

- reducing the cost of rework

Rigorously implement the Six Sigma improvement model: DMAIC (or DMEDVI)

Use a full range of statistical tools

Pursue perfection

Making Six Sigma work

Six Sigma focuses on how the company selects processes to improve and then schedules the processes to be improved.

Leaders begin by identifying the cost of poor quality. They focus on important processes and key issues affecting the company's business. They do not accept reworking, corrections, lost goods or services, inefficiencies, or lost productivity.

By prioritizing high-impact issues, leaders commission teams to focus on important problems with Black and Green Belt support. (*Note:* Some organizations have added an entry-level support person, called the White Belt.)

Employee training is fundamental to the Six Sigma processes. The significant training costs incurred should, however, be more than absorbed by the gains in profitability realized.

Figure 4.2	Master BB, BB, GB, WB

Title	Role
Process Owner / Champion	A person within executive or senior leadership with core accountability for the process to be improved. The improvement team is supported by and is ultimately accountable to the process owner.
Master Black Belt	Normally an external consultant, the Master Black Belt has deep expertise in six sigma tools and approaches. He or she consults with executive / senior leadership and internal black belts.
Black Belt	Black belts are internal experts whose full-time job is to support improvement teams and facilitate change. Black belts typically support up to four groups at the same time.
Green Belt	Green belts are typically middle managers or other key employees who receive training in six sigma tools and approaches and lead an improvement team working within their area of expertise / job responsibilities.
White Belt	White belts are improvement team members who are being developed in the tools and approaches.

Most successful implementations begin by engaging an outside consultant: a Master Black Belt. That person then develops Black, Green, and White Belts from within the organization's talent pool. Organizations that do not invest in a Master Black Belt at the beginning often have difficulty with their change processes and are less likely to have successful implementations.

After being trained, the Black, Green, and White Belts begin working on projects.

This Black to Green to White Belt hierarchy of improvement, talent, and focus is expensive. Therefore, it is not surprising that large organizations have an easier time covering the Six Sigma bill than do small ones.

| Figure 4.3 | **Leadership to Process Owner to improvement team** |

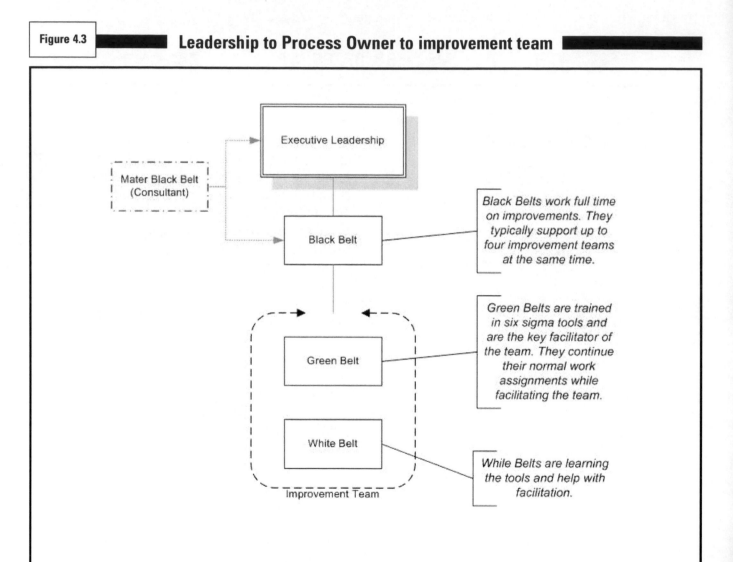

The prototypical "belt" structure for a Six Sigma company. A Master Black Belt consults from the outside, mainly working with executive leadership and internal Black Belts. One or more Black Belts are deployed to do nothing but work with improvement teams, and they can usually handle up to four teams at once. Within the team are Black Belts in training: the Green and White Belts. These employees typically maintain their normal work assignments.

Improvement teams consist of employees and are supported by Black Belts, Green Belts and sometimes, White Belts. The Process Owner is the person on the team who is responsible to senior leadership for the project and who works closely with the Black Belt. The Process Owner is expected to provide any support and resources the team needs.

Project selection

Selecting the right process to improve is the key to successful Six Sigma implementation. It requires that leaders truly understand company processes. Remember, a project is not considered a success unless the improvements realized positively impact the financial bottom line.

Question: How do you know a process is a candidate for improvement?
Answer: When it is not meeting customer needs.

Question: What do you mean by "customer needs"?
Answer: To answer this question, understand things such as how quickly the customer needs the product, what information the customer needs as part of the transaction, and at what point an error triggers the need for rework.

The improvement model—DMAIC

Although there are variations, the core Six Sigma improvement model includes the following steps:

1. **Define** (identification of the problem)
2. **Measure** (measuring the problem)
3. **Analyze** (identify the root cause of the problem)
4. **Improve** (mitigating the root cause)
5. **Control** (maintaining the gains)

The team, which consists of the Process Owner, the Belts, and staff who are responsible for the processes, usually meets each week to walk through the DMAIC process.

STEPS OF THE DMAIC PROCESS			
Breakthrough strategy	**Objective**	**Approach**	**Sample tools**
Define	✓ Identify key business issues ✓ Identify the problem	✓ Define goal and vision ✓ Identify customers' requirements ✓ Map the current process	✓ Affinity diagram ✓ Benchmarking ✓ Brainstorming ✓ Flow chart/ Process map ✓ GANTT chart
Measure	✓ Understand current perform-ance levels	✓ Gather data ✓ Measure performance	✓ Affinity diagram ✓ Check sheet ✓ Control charts/ Run chart ✓ Cycle time analysis ✓ Layout diagrams ✓ Pareto chart ✓ Responsibility flow chart ✓ Sigma ✓ Scatter diagram
Analyze	✓ Identify potential root causes	✓ Identify best practices ✓ Assess current performance	✓ Brainstorming ✓ Cause and effect ✓ Check sheets ✓ Control charts/ Run chart ✓ Cycle time analysis ✓ Failure Modes and Effects Analysis ✓ Flow chart/process map ✓ Histogram ✓ Pareto chart ✓ Scatter diagram ✓ Sigma

STEPS OF THE DMAIC PROCESS			
Breakthrough strategy	**Objective**	**Approach**	**Sample tools**
Improve	✓ Achieve breakthrough improvement	✓ Design new process ✓ Develop and establish plan for implementation	✓ Action plan worksheet ✓ Benchmarking ✓ Brainstorming ✓ Check sheet ✓ Control chart/ Run chart ✓ Cycle time analysis ✓ Failure Modes and Effects Analysis ✓ Flow chart/process maps ✓ GANTT chart ✓ Histogram ✓ Layout diagrams ✓ Pareto chart ✓ Responsibility flow chart ✓ Scatter diagram ✓ Standardized procedures
Control	✓ Establish standard procedures and measures ✓ Transform to how the day to day business is conducted	✓ Establish standard procedures and measures ✓ Monitor perform-ance and adjust as necessary	✓ Control charts/run charts ✓ Histogram ✓ Standardized procedures

Further information regarding tools can be obtained from a variety of sources (see p. 41).

Calculating Sigma

Calculating the sigma gives a numeric estimate of the overall quality of the process. Remember, the goal is six sigma. The steps in the calculation are as follows:

1. Calculate the total opportunities for a defect to occur
2. Calculate the defect rate
3. Calculate the defects per unit opportunity
4. Calculate the defects per million opportunities

Estimate the sigma value by using the results of step 4 and the sigma conversion table (Figure 4.4). The example that follows in Figure 4.4 demonstrates the sigma calculation of the timeliness of inpatient bed placement.

Figure 4.4

Sigma conversion table

Sigma	DPMO*	Yield (%)	Sigma	DPMO*	Yield (%)
6.0	3.4	99.99966	3.0	66,807	93.3
5.9	5.4	99.99946	2.9	80,757	91.9
5.8	8.5	99.99915	2.8	96,801	90.3
5.7	13	99.99866	2.7	115,070	88.5
5.6	21	99.9979	2.6	135,666	86.4
5.5	32	99.9968	2.5	158,655	84.1
5.4	48	99.9952	2.4	184,060	81.6
5.3	72	99.9928	2.3	211,855	78.8
5.2	108	99.9892	2.2	241,964	75.8
5.1	159	99.984	2.1	274,253	72.6
5.0	233	99.977	2.0	308,538	69.1
4.9	337	99.966	1.9	344,578	65.5
4.8	483	99.952	1.8	382,089	61.8
4.7	687	99.931	1.7	420,740	57.9
4.6	968	99.90	1.6	460,172	54.0
4.5	1,350	99.87	1.5	500,000	50.0
4.4	1,866	99.81	1.4	539,828	46.0
4.3	2,555	99.74	1.3	579,260	42.1
4.2	3,467	99.65	1.2	617,911	38.2
4.1	4,661	99.53	1.1	655,422	34.5
4.0	6,210	99.38	1.0	691,462	30.9
3.9	8,198	99.18	0.9	725,747	27.4
3.8	10,724	98.9	0.8	758,036	24.2
3.7	13,903	98.6	0.7	788,145	21.2
3.6	17,864	98.2	0.6	815,940	18.4
3.5	22,750	97.7	0.5	841,234	15.9
3.4	28,716	97.1	0.4	864,334	13.6
3.3	35,930	96.4	0.3	884,930	11.5
3.2	44,565	95.5	0.2	903,199	9.7
3.1	54,799	94.5	0.1	919,243	8.1

*DPMO = Defects per Million Opportunities.

SIX SIGMA CALCULATION OF TIMELINESS OF BED PLACEMENT

Step	In terms of bed placement	Result
1. Calculate the total opportunities for a defect to occur	The number of times a patient was to be placed in a hospital bed during the past month.	2,000
2. Calculate the defect rate	The number of times the patient was not placed in a room within 20 minutes after the room was ready and available during the past month.	200/2000 = 0.1
3. Calculate the defects per unit opportunity	There are 4 critical to quality (CTQ) steps in the bed availability process: Bed not available Bed not cleaned Bed cleaned, yet not released Bed released and not assigned Therefore, there are four potential defects (opportunities) per bed placement.	4/0.1=0.025
4. Calculate the defects per million opportunities	The number of failed bed placements per 1 million opportunities.	25,000
5. Estimate the sigma value by using the results of step 4 and the sigma conversion table to estimate the Six Sigma value.	Convert 25,000 defects per million opportunities to sigma using Figure 4.4.	3.4

Reporting to leadership

The DMAIC story: The project information must be packaged and reported to leadership. A frequently used tool is the DMAIC story, which summarizes the information from each step that the team completed and the measurements that support the outcome.

Scorecards measurements from the DMAIC story: Then place the measurements on a "Dash Board" or a "Scorecard" for ongoing communication of process performance. The measurement cycle is usually short and consistent.

Using Six Sigma on new processes

Although the Six Sigma approach works very well to improve existing processes, it really shines when it applied to the development of a new product.

This process is called "Design for Six Sigma" and uses a slightly modified model: DMEDVI. The steps include the following:

- Define
- Measure
- Explore
- Design
- Validate
- Implement

As in improvement projects, design efforts are led by the Master Black Belts and Black Belts.

Healthcare applications

The application of Six Sigma in other industries, including some service organizations, has been successful in increasing profitability and quality. It works for the *business* practices of healthcare just well as it works in these other industries. Using Six Sigma to improve *clinical* processes, however, has proven more difficult for a number of reasons:

- The relationship between a clinical process and the bottom line may be indirect or obscure
- Clinical processes tend to be very complex and interdependent with other processes
- Data to measure clinical processes are often difficult to obtain

Despite these problems, however, Six Sigma can and has worked to improve clinical as well as business processes.

Six Sigma structure

The following are "typical" roles within a Six Sigma structure. These roles are evolving in healthcare and some smaller institutions may find it possible to discover more efficient, less costly structure. However, the structure below has a proven track record of success in other industries.

- **Champions** or **Sponsors** ensure that the project stays on track. They usually have high-level managerial responsibility for the process the project. They typically are held accountable for the project's success. They regularly monitor the program results and accomplishments.

- **Master Black Belts** are consultants (internal or external) that serve as coaches and mentors to the Black Belts. They are true experts in the Six Sigma analytical tools. They also serve as an organizational change agent by promoting the use of Six Sigma methods and solutions. Master Black Belts have proven to be important to the overall success of organizations' transitions to Six Sigma.

- **Black Belts** are trained to be change agents and are proficient in the use of Six Sigma tools. Their full-time responsibility is the education, guidance, and management of project teams. They are focused on the teams to which they are assigned, rather than on the overall implementation of Six Sigma.

- **Green Belts** assist the Black Belt in larger projects and can act as team leaders for smaller scale efforts. They are often Black Belts in training. They work within their department on a regular basis and get time to work on the team's efforts with the Black Belt. Their training is similar to that of Black Belt; however, they may have less experience and time to devote to the project.

- **White Belts** are entry-level Six Sigma facilitators who have received some training in tools and approaches. As they develop, they apply problem-solving skills within their area of responsibility.

- **Team Members** form the core work group of the project and typically are employees who participate in the process under study daily. Those who have specialized knowledge may be ad-hoc team members.

- **Senior Leaders** must be part of the improvement by sharing in the responsibility of the project and the overall implementation. Ultimately, the success or failure of the effort will rest, in large part, on the level of focus and commitment by Senior Leaders.

Close attention to the Six Sigma structure seems to be play a very important role in the success of the effort.

Each person in the organization must focus on his or her respective area of responsibility. For instance, during the measurement stage,

- leaders focus on the bottom line and profits
- operations leaders are responsible for measuring cost relative to their area of function

Black Belts are responsible for measurements and assessing their functions. They assess the gaps in performance, how processes affect other processes, and how to begin to develop the necessary breakthroughs.

SIX SIGMA RESOURCES

Michael Brassard and Diane Ritter, Sailing *Through Six Sigma.*

Mikel Harry, PhD, and Richard Schroeder, *Six Sigma.*

www.sixsigmamainstreet.com/home.asp.

CASE STUDY	SIX SIGMA IMPROVEMENT EXAMPLE: SCHEDULING IN LABOR AND DELIVERY

Project selection

A scheduling process in labor and delivery might be selected as a Six Sigma improvement project for any of the following reasons:

- The hospital is concerned about the amount of overtime use.
- The hospital is concerned that it may be successfully sued in a "bad baby" case related to lack of experienced nurses. (Damages in such cases range from about $250,000 to millions of dollars.)
- A professional liability case settled in the past focused leadership's attention on the unit.
- Low patient or physician satisfaction is impacting volume or payer mix.

Theorizing a return to the bottom line from professional liability cases that are not filed is difficult, but it is a "leap of faith" most leaders are prepared to take. In an ideal world, the return would be expressed in terms of decreased malpractice premiums or reserves, but we know the world is often less than ideal.

Likewise, we understand that there is a relationship between satisfaction and volume and a similar relationship between satisfaction and payer mix. However, like decreased liability risks, it is difficult to put a cost per defect impact due to decreased satisfaction on the bottom line.

Therefore, increased satisfaction alone or decreased professional liability risk alone would not be sufficient to justify selection of the project following a strict Six Sigma approach.

Defining the measurable problem

So, what defects are we trying to avoid and what is the cost per defect? In the labor and delivery example, the defect was a shift that lacked sufficient nursing coverage due to a scheduling error.

We assume that the defect (i.e., insufficient nurse coverage due to scheduling problems) occurred between one and four times a week, creating overtime costs to the organization. The average cost of the scheduling error was $70 an hour, and the effect lasted from 12–48 hours, putting the total

SIX SIGMA IMPROVEMENT EXAMPLE: SCHEDULING IN LABOR AND DELIVERY (CONT.)

cost per error between $840 and $3,360. The annual cost of such scheduling errors could cost the organization between $43,680 and $174,720. Therefore, reducing this defect would put money back on the bottom line in an immediate and tangible way.

Putting Six Sigma to work

An essential concept of Six Sigma is the importance of the customer. This is called the voice of the customer, or VOC.

Customers of healthcare (patients and physicians) do not expect or tolerate defects. They expect that things will go smoothly and that the patient care unit will be staffed appropriately. For example, patients expect the birth process to be safe and that staff and physicians will protect them from adverse events. The customer requirement in this instance may look like this:

VOICE OF CUSTOMER				
Customer says	Meaning to our business	Critical to quality name	Customer requirement	Critical to quality measure
I expect the staff to be able to help me	Provide staff who are able to help	Staff available	Staff courteous and competent	Cost is contained
I expect a healthy baby	Prevent poor baby outcomes	No adverse events	Baby is healthy	

Calculating baseline sigma

Here are the "givens":

- There are from one to four shifts per week during which a scheduling error results in either overtime or short staffing.
- The total number of shifts per week is 280.

SIX SIGMA IMPROVEMENT EXAMPLE: SCHEDULING IN LABOR AND DELIVERY (CONT.)

Step 1: Calculate the total opportunities for a defect to occur.

For the sake of simplicity, we assume that there is only one way for a defect to occur: the shift is not covered. Therefore, the total number of opportunities for the defect to occur is once per shift per week, or 280.

Step 2: Calculate the defect rate (defects per unit)

Between one and four of the 280 weekly shifts are not covered. The defect rate per shift therefore ranges between 1/280 (0.0036) and 4/280 (0.0143). We take the higher of these numbers, which is the true reliability of the scheduling system.

Step 3: Calculate defects per opportunity

If there were four ways we could make an error in scheduling, we would divide the raw defect rate by 4. If there were two ways, we divide by 2.

For the sake of simplicity, we assume that there is only one type of shift-scheduling error. Therefore, the defects per opportunity are the same as the defects per unit (shift), or 0.0143.

Step 4: Calculate defects per million opportunities

Multiply 0.0143 by a million (10^6) (move the decimal point six places to the right), or 14,300 defects per million opportunities.

Step 5: Estimate the sigma from the conversion chart

Looking at the chart in Figure 4.4, we see that 14,300 defects per million opportunities translates to approximately 3.7σ . . . a long way from our goal of 6σ.

Also from the conversion table in Figure 4.4, you'll notice a "yield" of 98.6%.

You should avail yourself of a "six sigma calculator" if you'll be doing this type of calculation frequently. Check out sites such as *www*.sixsigma.com for possible tools, or take the time to reduce the math to an easy spreadsheet.

Note that the reliability of the scheduling system almost 99%. Yet it still should be improved.

<table>
<tr><td>**CASE STUDY**</td><td>**SIX SIGMA IMPROVEMENT EXAMPLE: SCHEDULING IN LABOR AND DELIVERY (CONT.)**</td></tr>
</table>

We find it far easier to see the progress from 3.7σ to 4.7σ toward 6σ than to track yield as it inches from 98.6% toward 99.99966%. We therefore understand the potential attraction and power of the Six Sigma mindset.

Figure 4.5

Tracking sigma v. yield

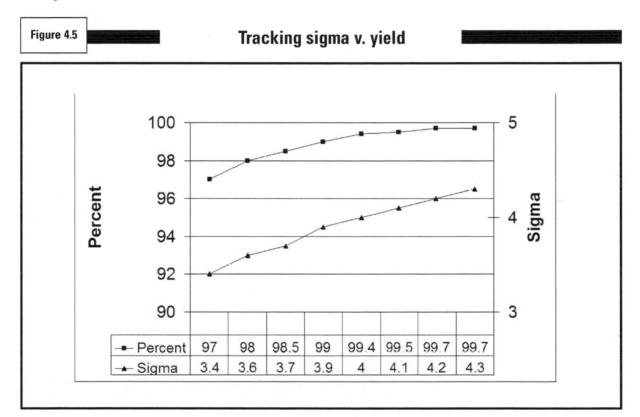

Percent	97	98	98.5	99	99.4	99.5	99.7	99.7
Sigma	3.4	3.6	3.7	3.9	4	4.1	4.2	4.3

Project support

The labor and delivery team will have a lot of work to do to reduce the number of scheduling errors (defects) per week. If the team is able to reduce the number of scheduling errors to one every other week, the process will perform at 4.19σ with a Yield of 99.64%.

Because this is one of the first Six Sigma processes the hospital undertakes, leadership enlists the aid of a Master Black Belt consultant.

The project becomes one of the four assigned to a full-time Black Belt.

CASE STUDY	**SIX SIGMA IMPROVEMENT EXAMPLE: SCHEDULING IN LABOR AND DELIVERY (CONT.)**

A Green Belt is assigned to assist in the project. It is his or her only project for now, but the Green Belt has other duties within the organization.

A Champion, the nurse manager of labor and delivery, is selected.

Project launch

Forming the team

Team members must have good working knowledge of the process that is to be improved. They must be willing to change the process. They also must be smart and have the energy to participate. The selection of the team members is as critical as selecting the Black and Green Belts. The organization that selects people who are not seen as influential within their work unit may doom the project, since they are the same people who will be going back to the unit to discuss and help implement the solutions.

The people selected to work on the labor and delivery scheduling project included a staff nurse from the day shift, a staff nurse from the night shift, a shift manager, the manager over the labor and delivery unit, and the hospital's nurse executive. The unit manager had just finished Green Belt training. The Sponsor in this case was the nurse executive. The Black Belt was a full-time employee from inside the organization who had access to a Master Black Belt for assistance as needed.

Developing the charter

The charter is the reason for doing the project. It guides the team. It should have the purpose, goal, and scope of the project. Usually charters are written by the Sponsor and then are refined by the team. When the charter is refined, it must go back for review by the Sponsor to ensure that the intent of the project is on track.

SIX SIGMA IMPROVEMENT EXAMPLE: SCHEDULING IN LABOR AND DELIVERY (CONT.)

LABOR AND DELIVERY SCHEDULING CHARTER

The project: "Reduce the number of scheduling errors"

Leader: Labor and delivery manager

Black Belt: Assigned from consulting firm

Green Belt: Medical surgical nursing director

Project start date: XX

Project end date: XX

Cost of poor quality: Between $43,680.00 and $174,720.00 annually, without consideration of increase liability or decreased satisfaction. Team Members: Assigned

Champion/Sponsor: Nurse Executive

Process importance: Nurses are to be scheduled to care for the patients

Process problem: Scheduling errors have resulted in either overtime costs or working with less nurses than was scheduled for the patient census.

Project goals: Reduce scheduling errors by 75%, with a savings between $32,760 and $130,629 annually. Reduce the number of no shows by the staff by 75%.

Training the team

Training is ongoing for the team. It can take from one to many weeks depending on the complexity of the project. The team may receive some of the training in a classroom setting; however most training occurs as the team works through its process. This training is provided by the Black Belt assigned to the team.

DMAIC

The DMAIC problem-solving process, described earlier, is not necessarily linear. Teams often go back and forth to the various steps of the process as new information becomes available.

D—Define the problem

A schedule request system is in place to provide staff nurses with input regarding their schedule. However, there are times when a nurse does not present for duty due to an error in the scheduling process. Assigned staff members who do not report to duty frequently trigger the need for overtime, which costs the organization money that is not an added value.

Such scheduling errors arise from a variety of sources.

M—Measure

A fundamental step to improving any process is to develop a way to measure the critical parts. In this case we want to measure the flaws: the scheduling errors. Therefore, scheduling errors are counted in terms of frequency and the underlying reason (or subprocess) associated with them.

Potential measures of the problem were number of

- overtime hours due to scheduling errors
- scheduling errors categorized by the cause of the error
- scheduling errors that resulted in a "no show" categorized by the cause of the error

---

THE MATHEMATICS OF A SYSTEM

Organizational processes or operational systems can be viewed in a mathematical model with inputs (x) to functions (f) contributing to the outcome (Y). In other words, the outcome (Y) is a result of an indefinite number of functions (f) or subprocesses, each with its own input (x).

$$Y = \Sigma f_{1-n}(x)$$

Scheduling Error with a "no show" (Y) = the sum of subprocesses that contributed to the scheduling error [f(x)]

A—Analyze

The team's next step is to identify all of the subprocesses that contribute to scheduling error and then determine the root cause(s) of these flaws in the system.

<table>
<tr><td>

CASE STUDY

</td><td>

SIX SIGMA IMPROVEMENT EXAMPLE: SCHEDULING IN LABOR AND DELIVERY (CONT.)

</td></tr>
</table>

The team uses a Failure Modes and Effects Analysis (FMEA) to understand all of the potential contributors to the error. The first step was to create flow diagram of the process as it was performing (see Figure 4.6).

Figure 4.6   **L and D scheduling flow diagram**

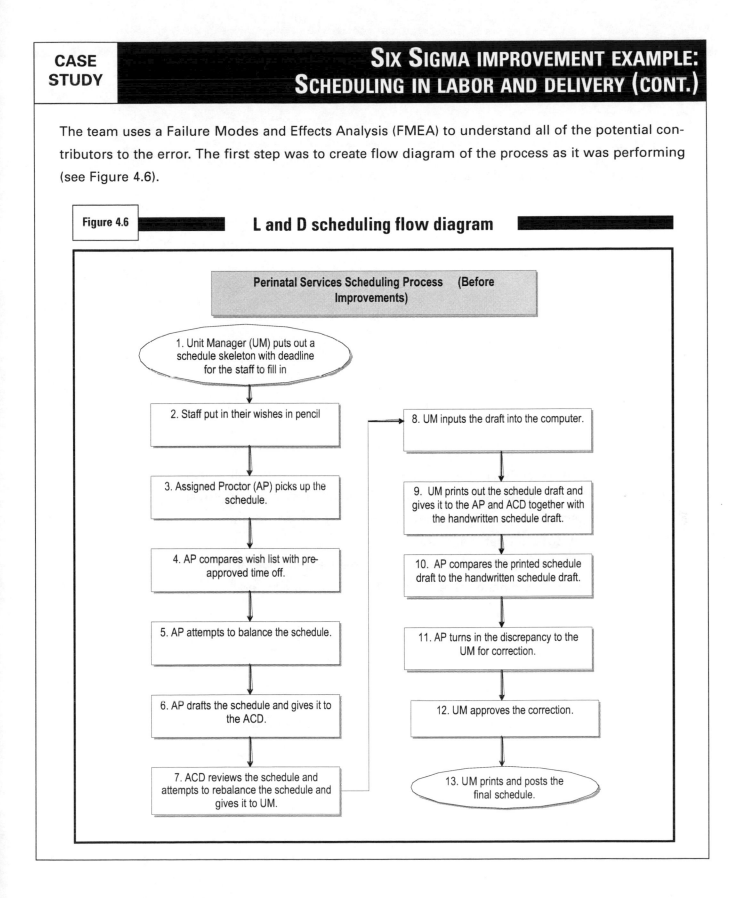

Perinatal Services Scheduling Process   (Before Improvements)

1. Unit Manager (UM) puts out a schedule skeleton with deadline for the staff to fill in

2. Staff put in their wishes in pencil

3. Assigned Proctor (AP) picks up the schedule.

4. AP compares wish list with pre-approved time off.

5. AP attempts to balance the schedule.

6. AP drafts the schedule and gives it to the ACD.

7. ACD reviews the schedule and attempts to rebalance the schedule and gives it to UM.

8. UM inputs the draft into the computer.

9. UM prints out the schedule draft and gives it to the AP and ACD together with the handwritten schedule draft.

10. AP compares the printed schedule draft to the handwritten schedule draft.

11. AP turns in the discrepancy to the UM for correction.

12. UM approves the correction.

13. UM prints and posts the final schedule.

CASE STUDY	SIX SIGMA IMPROVEMENT EXAMPLE: SCHEDULING IN LABOR AND DELIVERY (CONT.)

After flow charting the scheduling process, the various known, and potential "failure modes" [f(x)] are identified and their effects ranked. The frequency of occurrence of these various failure modes may then be measured, feeding back to the previous (Measure) step.

Under the supervision and guidance of the Black Belt, the team reviewed the scheduling data collected by the unit manager. As the team assessed the data and conducted its FMEA, it discovered several issues:

- Deadline was not met to put out the "skeleton" schedule
- Computer is down
- Printer is down
- No one knows how to print the schedule
- New employees are not on the skeleton schedule, and staff forget their vacation
- Skeleton lost in the unit
- Staff members fail to put in their wishes/requests
- Staff members don't put in the time that correlates with their commitment or status
- Staff members give themselves days off without obtaining prior approval
- Staff members write in the wrong date on the schedule request form
- The manager does not get the information
- Staff members are unwilling to change requested days to cover the unit
- Schedule requests are handwritten rather than computer entered

The effects of these potential causes were rated by their likelihood to lead to a system failure (following the FMEA method).

I—Improve

A prioritized action plan (based on the risk that the failure mode contributed to a "no show") was developed and implemented.

Improvements included the following:

- The unit manager developed written instructions for printing the skeleton schedule.
- Assistant managers were trained on how to print the skeleton schedule.
- The unit manager routinely published/posted the skeleton schedule indicating the pre-approved vacations.
- Staff members who were assigned to work received the skeleton schedule one week prior to the two-week schedule period.
- Vacations were written in red ink.
- Photocopies of the schedule were made prior to releasing it to the staff.
- Time-off forms were left in a designated place on the unit.
- The unit manager ensured that the schedule was balanced based on the requests received.
- A new computer was purchased to support the scheduling application.
- The Sponsor and senior leadership were apprised of the action plan and performance results ongoing.

| Figure 4.7 | **FMEA for L and D staffing** |

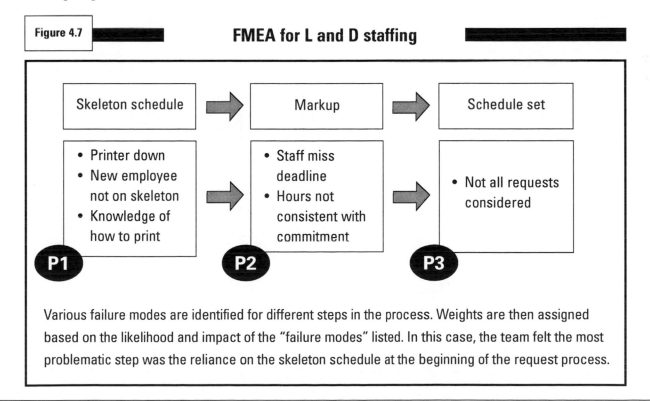

Various failure modes are identified for different steps in the process. Weights are then assigned based on the likelihood and impact of the "failure modes" listed. In this case, the team felt the most problematic step was the reliance on the skeleton schedule at the beginning of the request process.

CASE STUDY	SIX SIGMA IMPROVEMENT EXAMPLE: SCHEDULING IN LABOR AND DELIVERY (CONT.)

C—Control

The team continued to measure the number of scheduling errors made each month and the amount of overtime as a result of a scheduling error. Implementation of proposed actions and their impact on scheduling continues to be tracked.

Results

Scheduling errors were reduced to one in every four weeks. The new sigma was calculated to be 4.62, with a yield of 99.91%.

The project resulted in a reduction of overtime due to scheduling errors to $10,040.00 per year (annualized projection), representing annual savings between $33,640.00 and $164,648.00.

The costs associated with a "bad baby" liability claims and satisfaction are not calculated into this saving. However, the number of adverse occurrences, satisfaction and claims should continue to be tracked as ongoing indicators of aggregate labor and delivery processes.

The frequency of scheduling errors was placed on the unit scorecard to ensure ongoing control (maintaining the gains).

CASE STUDY

SIX SIGMA IMPROVEMENT EXAMPLE: SCHEDULING IN LABOR AND DELIVERY (CONT.)

Figure 4.8

Labor and delivery scheduling FMEA
FMEA team start-up worksheet (steps 1 & 2)

FMEA Project Name:	FMEA Perinatal Services Self Scheduling
Facilitator	LManigbas, RN
Team Leader:	C. Horton, RN, Director, Perinatal Services
Date FMEA Started (to be started):	May 5, 2004
Team Sponsors:	Perinatal PI & RM Committee
Team Members: (Step 2)	◆ N. Abe, RN, ACD ◆ Y. Barillas, RN, ACD ◆ C. Boone, RN, ACD ◆ E. Go, RN, ACD ◆ T. Magcalas, RN, ACD ◆ D. Mihara, RN, ACD ◆ S. Smith, RN, ACD ◆ J. Rodriguez, RN, ACD ◆ T. Williams, RN, ACD ◆ E. Jones, Unit Manager ◆ L&D Staff

Team Leader Questions:

1.	Are all affected areas represented?	Yes
2.	Are different levels and types of knowledge represented on the team?	Yes
3.	Who will maintain the records?	L&D Department Administrator or Designee

FMEA Team Project Boundaries (Step 1):

1.	Project Purpose (including a description of the process under review):	To decrease the "No show" rate in L&D To decrease % of overtime in L&D
2.	What aspects of the FMEA is the team responsible for?	✓ FMEA Analysis ✓ Recommendations for Improvement ✓ Implementation of Improvements (except for actions requiring budget approval)
3.	Reporting Body(s): Who will receive progress reports?	Perinatal PI & RM Committee Medical Center Operations Team
4.	Project Deadlines:	August 2004
5.	What is the process if the team needs to expand beyond these boundaries?	Need to present a business case for budget approval

CASE STUDY

SIX SIGMA IMPROVEMENT EXAMPLE: SCHEDULING IN LABOR AND DELIVERY (CONT.)

Figure 4.9

FMEA worksheet for labor and delivery scheduling (steps 3–11)

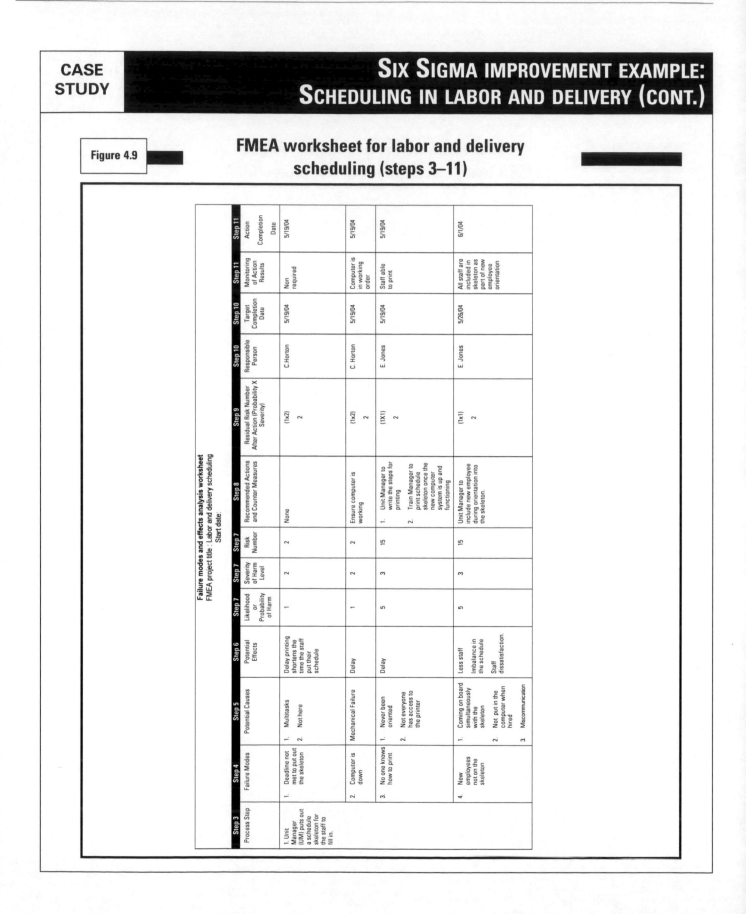

Failure modes and effects analysis worksheet
FMEA project title : Labor and delivery scheduling
Start date:

Step 3 Process Step	Step 4 Failure Modes	Step 5 Potential Causes	Step 6 Potential Effects	Step 7 Likelihood or Probability of Harm	Step 7 Severity of Harm Level	Step 7 Risk Number	Step 8 Recommended Actions and Counter Measures	Step 9 Residual Risk Number After Action (Probability X Severity)	Step 10 Responsible Person	Step 10 Target Completion Date	Step 11 Monitoring of Action Results	Step 11 Action Completion Date
1. Unit Manager (UM) puts out a skeleton schedule for the staff to fill in.	1. Deadline not met to put out the skeleton	1. Multitasks 2. Not here	Delay printing shortens the time the staff put their schedule	1	2	2	None	(1x2) 2	C. Horton	5/19/04	Non required	5/19/04
	2. Computer is down	Mechanical Failure	Delay	1	2	2	Ensure computer is working	(1x2) 2	C. Horton	5/19/04	Computer is in working order	5/19/04
	3. No one knows how to print	1. Never been oriented 2. Not everyone has access to the printer	Delay	5	3	15	1. Unit Manager to write the steps for printing 2. Train Manager to print schedule skeleton once the new computer system is up and functioning	(1X1) 2	E. Jones	5/19/04	Staff able to print	5/19/04
	4. New employees not on the skeleton	1. Coming on board simultaneously with the skeleton 2. Not put in the computer when hired 3. Miscommunication	Less staff Imbalance in the schedule Staff dissatisfaction.	5	3	15	Unit Manager to include new employee during orientation into the skeleton.	(1x1) 2	E. Jones	5/26/04	All staff are included in skeleton as part of new employee orientation	6/1/04

CASE STUDY

SIX SIGMA IMPROVEMENT EXAMPLE: SCHEDULING IN LABOR AND DELIVERY (CONT.)

Figure 4.9

FMEA worksheet for labor and delivery scheduling (steps 3–11) (cont.)

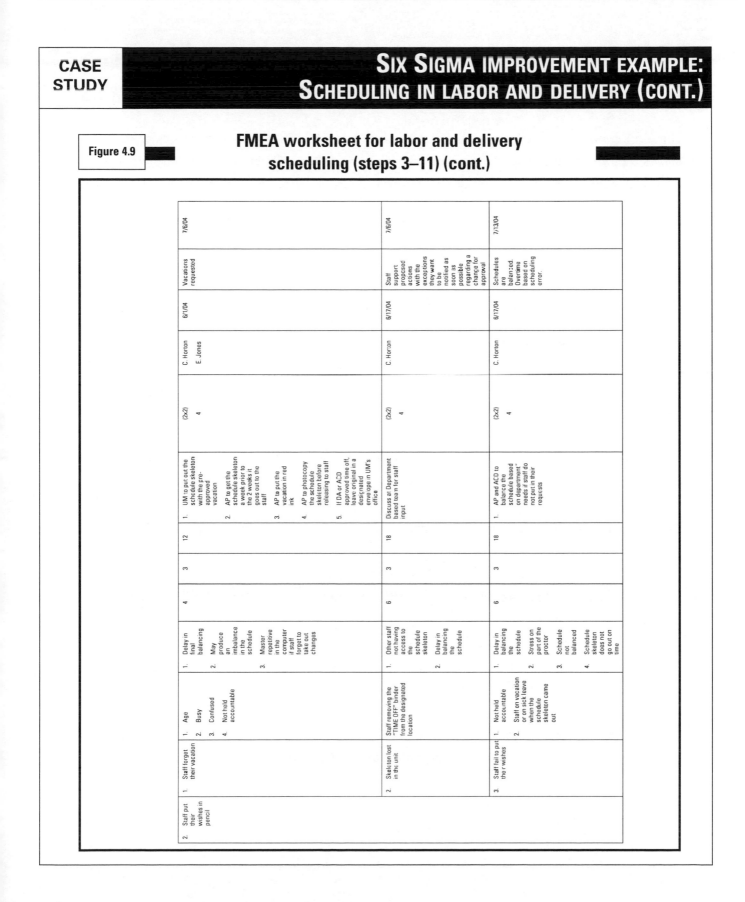

SIX SIGMA IMPROVEMENT EXAMPLE: PATIENT FALLS

The Six Sigma model views operational processes mathematically. This mathematical approach allows a more precise view of the process so it can be better understood and controlled—that is, so we can distinguish true change (hopefully improvement) from chance variations in performance.

This scenario focuses on a problem that most hospitals have been struggling with for years: patient falls. However, it will view this common issue through the lens of Six Sigma. We assume that leadership has already allocated Black Belt and other resources and is in the process of changing the organization's way of thinking.

Project selection

The first step was establishing the link between decreasing patient falls and the hospital's financial bottom line. Falls have primary, secondary, and tertiary cost streams:

The **primary** costs of falls are those associated with the post-fall assessment to determine the extent of the patient's injury, if any (imaging studies, physician examinations, etc.).

Secondary costs are those associated with treating patient injuries, including extending the patient's stay.

The **tertiary** costs of falls are payments to settle general and professional liability claims.

Secondary and tertiary costs are highly variable and, most would argue, not *tangible* enough to serve as the basis for a Six Sigma project. Therefore, the hospital fixed its sights on the primary (diagnostic) costs of falls.

The average **primary** (assessment) cost of each fall at this hospital is $1,000. There are about 12 falls per month estimated to cost the organization $12,000 a month or $144,000 in primary costs each year. We also suspect that the secondary and tertiary costs, although intangible for the sake of this project, are significantly higher.

The rigor with which Six Sigma looks to tangible cost savings during project selection distinguishes it from traditional TQM and later models, such as Lean Thinking and rapid cycle testing. Even though these other models focus on data-driven, tangible improvements, they are not necessarily linked to demonstrable short-term financial improvements. A rule of thumb is that a Six Sigma project should save the organization at least $250,000.

The total primary costs of patient falls ($144,000) was less than the total savings for a typical Six Sigma project ($250,000). However, it was known that the tertiary costs (settlements) for falls had been $500,000 for the previous year, with unknown secondary costs (direct cost of treating injuries due to falls) of poor quality. In all, patient falls seemed to have excellent potential for a Six Sigma project.

VOC AND CTQ

VOC stands for voice of the customer, who is envisioned to be at the table and heard loudly in any definition of quality and in all improvement projects.

Decreasing falls is definitely in tune with the VOC.

The patient does not expect to fall victim to avoidable injuries due to a fall.

The Joint Commission on Accreditation of Healthcare Organizations, another important customer, recently adopted patient falls as one of its National Patient Safety Goals.

By listening to the VOC, the project team can learn about those elements of their product that are critical to quality (CTQ).

The organization clearly heard the VOC say that preventing avoidable injuries was CTQ. It is therefore a good target for improvement.

CASE STUDY	SIX SIGMA IMPROVEMENT EXAMPLE: PATIENT FALLS (CONT.)

Calculating baseline sigma

Here are the "givens":

> There are 12 falls in an average month.
> There are 3000 patient-days in an average month.

Step 1: Calculate the total opportunities for a defect to occur.

For the sake of simplicity we assume that there is only one way for a defect to occur: the patient has one opportunity to fall during each day of their stay. Therefore, the total number of opportunities for the patient to fall is equal to the number of patient days, or **3000**.

Step 2: Calculate the defect rate (defects per unit)

There are 12 falls per 3000 units or patient days. Therefore, the defect rate is 12/3,000 or 0.004.

Step 3: Calculate defects per opportunity

Because we've assumed only one opportunity per patient day, the defects per opportunity is the same as the defect rate, or 0.004.

Step 4: Calculate defects per million opportunities

Multiplying the defect by 1 million shows a rate of 4,000 defects (falls) per million opportunities.

Step 5: Estimate the "sigma" from the conversion chart

Looking at the chart in Figure 4.4, we see that 4,000 defects per million opportunities translates to approximately 4.15σ. This is actually not bad, especially given the conservative assumption about the number of opportunities to fall each day. However, is it good enough? We don't think so. Also, from the conversion table in Figure 4.4, you'll notice a "yield" of 99.6%.

The team will have a lot of work to do to reduce the number of falls per month. If the team is able to reduce the number of falls to two per month, the sigma will be 4.709, with a yield of 99.93%. If they are able to reduce the fall rate to two per year, then the sigma will be 5.365 with a yield of 99.99%.

Remember, 6 is twice 3, but 6σ is about 20,000 times better than 3σ. Performance at 6σ is near absolute perfection, or about 3.5 defects per million opportunities.

Project support

The organization selects the project and enlists the aid of a Master Black Belt, a Black Belt, and a Green Belt to assist in the project. It also selects a Champion or a Sponsor.

Project launch

Forming the team

Team members must have good working knowledge of the process that is to be improved. They must also be willing to change the process. They must be smart and have energy to participate. The selection of the team members is as critical as selecting the Black and Green Belts. The organization that selects people who are not seen as influential within their work unit may doom the project, since they are the very same people who will be going back to the unit to discuss and help implement the solutions.

In this scenario, the people selected were a staff nurse from the day shift, a staff nurse from the night shift, a clinical instructor, a shift manager, a unit clerk, the director of the units, and the nurse executive. The director of the units had just received the Green Belt training. The Sponsor in this case was the nurse executive, who wanted to be part of the team because of the project implications for overall nursing practice. The Black Belt was hired from a consulting firm and had access to a Master Black Belt for assistance as needed.

Developing the charter

This provides the reason for doing the project. It serves as a guide for the team. It should have the purpose, goal, and scope of the project, which usually are written by the Champion and then are refined by the team. It is important that, when the Charter is refined, it goes back for review by the Champion to ensure that the intent of the project is on track as desired by the Champion.

SIX SIGMA IMPROVEMENT EXAMPLE: PATIENT FALLS (CONT.)

Training the team

Training is ongoing for the team. It can take from one to many weeks, depending on the complexity of the project. The team may receive some of the training in a classroom setting; however, most of it is seen in the real work application of the team. This training is provided by the assigned Black Belt to the team.

PATIENT FALLS PROJECT CHARTER

The project: "Reduce the number of patients who fall in the medical surgical units"

Leader: Medical surgical nursing director

Black Belt: Assigned from consulting firm

Green Belt: Medical surgical nursing director

Project start date: XX

Project end date: XX

Cost of poor quality: more than $600,000 (tangible and intangible)

Team members: Day-shift staff nurse, night-shift staff nurse, clinical instructor, shift manager, unit clerk, the unit manager, and nurse executive

Champion/Sponsor: Nurse executive

Process importance: Patient is falling and is being injured while entrusted to our care

Process problem: The fall prevention process has not provided consistent results

Project goals: Reduce medical/surgical falls by 50%, with a savings of $72,000 in tangible primary costs and at least $300,000 overall

<table>
<tr><td>**CASE STUDY**</td><td>**SIX SIGMA IMPROVEMENT EXAMPLE: PATIENT FALLS (CONT.)**</td></tr>
</table>

DMAIC

D—Define the problem

Patients are assessed for the risk of falling when they come into the organization. However, the risk assessment is not always accurate in predicting a fall, and the assessment does not always trigger an intervention that prevented the fall.

Figure 4.10

Ishikawa or cause and effect diagram for falls

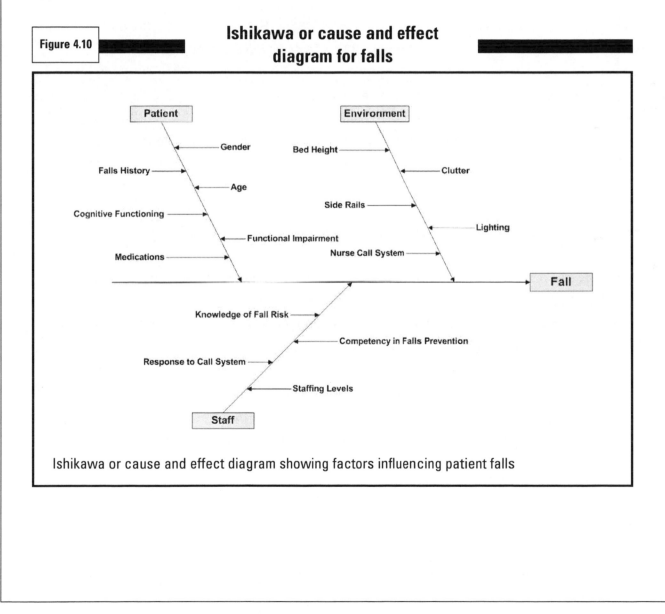

Ishikawa or cause and effect diagram showing factors influencing patient falls

SIX SIGMA IMPROVEMENT EXAMPLE: PATIENT FALLS (CONT.)

M—Measure

Although it is possible to measure assessments and interventions, the ultimate CTQ factor (listening to the VOC) is the number of falls.

The severity of falls is another potential measure, along with a host of other variables.

A—Analyze

The team, under the supervision and guidance of the Black Belt, reviewed the fall data collected by the risk manager. During the assessment of the data, they discovered the following:

- Falls associated with toileting during the evening and mid-morning hours had the most injuries
- Men and women had equal chances of falling
- There was a direct correlation between patient age and likelihood of fallings
- Those with cognitive impairment and a history of a prior fall more often fell with resulting injuries

The falls-prevention policy called for a number of interventions, such as

- placing the patient near the nursing station (which happened for most of the patients who fell)
- making rounds at least every two hours for at-risk patients
- placing a sticker on the assignment board that the patient was assessed as at risk for a fall
- including the risk rating as part of the activity record
- use of a patient teaching record that identifies whether the patient is at risk for a fall
- creating queues for the nurse to provide orientation to the patient and family to the room and environment at the time of admission and as needed if there is alternation in mentation
- keeping articles, such as call lights, urinals, tissues, and telephones within easy reach of the patients in bed or up in a chair
- keeping the room free of hazards (clutter)
- identifying that the patient is at risk in the problem goal list
- answering call lights promptly
- assisting patients to the bathroom in the early morning, after meals, and at bedtime
- ensuring that the bed is in lowest position possible

| CASE STUDY | **SIX SIGMA IMPROVEMENT EXAMPLE: PATIENT FALLS (CONT.)** |

The following factors were NOT addressed:

- Consideration of the use of a sitter if the patient was a fall risk
- Consideration of the use of a vest restraint (restraint in general was discouraged by the organization)
- A method of communication to others in the healthcare team about the patient's risk of falling

In assessment, the physical environment was not found to be a contributing factor in those falls with injuries.

In addition, there was a prevailing attitude that all patients were at risk for falls and that, therefore, they could not be prevented.

The team also pointed out that fall reduction had not been made a priority by hospital leadership.

Finally, when the patient was taken to other units, there was not a consistent system for communicating that the patient was at risk for falls.

I—Improve

Articles published on the prevention of falls lacked hard data about what worked and what didn't.

Some literature suggested that improved toileting interventions for at-risk patient may reduce falls.

JCAHO's National Patient Safety Goal addressing falls asked the hospital to

- include the cognitive or hemodynamic effects of medications in patient fall assessments
- consider the use of low beds and bed alarms for at-risk patients
- reduce use of full length rails

The team recommended the following to leadership (remember, in this case the sponsor was on the team; had that not been the case, the sponsor would have received regular reports from the Black Belt and Green Belt regarding the process of the team).

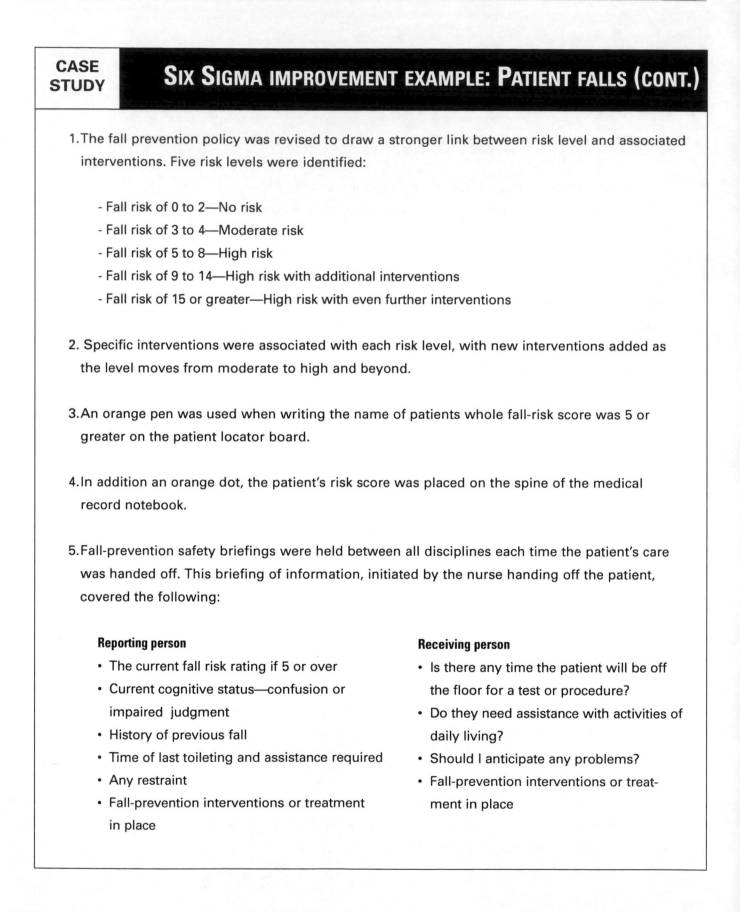

| CASE STUDY | SIX SIGMA IMPROVEMENT EXAMPLE: PATIENT FALLS (CONT.) |

1. The fall prevention policy was revised to draw a stronger link between risk level and associated interventions. Five risk levels were identified:

   - Fall risk of 0 to 2—No risk
   - Fall risk of 3 to 4—Moderate risk
   - Fall risk of 5 to 8—High risk
   - Fall risk of 9 to 14—High risk with additional interventions
   - Fall risk of 15 or greater—High risk with even further interventions

2. Specific interventions were associated with each risk level, with new interventions added as the level moves from moderate to high and beyond.

3. An orange pen was used when writing the name of patients whole fall-risk score was 5 or greater on the patient locator board.

4. In addition an orange dot, the patient's risk score was placed on the spine of the medical record notebook.

5. Fall-prevention safety briefings were held between all disciplines each time the patient's care was handed off. This briefing of information, initiated by the nurse handing off the patient, covered the following:

Reporting person
- The current fall risk rating if 5 or over
- Current cognitive status—confusion or impaired judgment
- History of previous fall
- Time of last toileting and assistance required
- Any restraint
- Fall-prevention interventions or treatment in place

Receiving person
- Is there any time the patient will be off the floor for a test or procedure?
- Do they need assistance with activities of daily living?
- Should I anticipate any problems?
- Fall-prevention interventions or treatment in place

6. Management staff members are also expected to make rounds at least once each shift to help staff with assessments and interventions. In addition to providing substantive assistance, doing so communicates the importance of falls prevention throughout the nursing organization.

C—Control

The team continued to measure the number of falls per month.

These measures and other falls issues were communicated to staff during management rounds and regular patient safety briefings.

Results

Falls were reduced to **four per month, a 75% reduction.**

The revised sigma was 4.5 with a yield of 99.87% compared to the earlier performance of 4.15. Although this may seem a small change, improvement becomes difficult the closer one gets to perfection. Moving from 99.6% to 99.87% yield is, in fact, an important move forward.

There were no falls associated with an injury that required additional length of stay, or additional treatment, other than the initial assessment.

There were no cash payouts to settle falls claims (compared to $500,000 in the past).

The primary (assessment) costs were reduced from $12,000 per month to $2,000 per month, for a savings of $100,000 per year.

CHAPTER FIVE

LEAN THINKING

LEAN THINKING

ELEVATOR DESCRIPTION OF LEAN THINKING

Quick: You have a two-floor ride in an elevator with your CEO and medical director and they want to know about Lean Thinking.

Lean Thinking is a systematic approach to the identification and elimination of waste in the production of products or delivery of services.

Lean Thinking, pioneered by Toyota, is doing more with less waste—that is, fewer activities that do not add value to the customer—while providing customers **what** they want **when** they want it. Lean Thinking identifies and eliminates waste. It is a rigorous approach to the identification of "non-value-added" activities.

Listening to the VOC

Like Six Sigma, Lean Thinking is not about convincing the customer to accept services or products that an organization wants to provide. Instead, it's about listening to the voice of the customer (VOC) and delivering what it wants.

In the past, many organizations have allowed the person providing the service or product to define quality rather than allowing quality to be defined by the needs and wants of external and internal customers.

"No problem," you think. "From now on, we'll just let the customer define quality." But it's not as easy as it sounds.

Customers usually make choices among those products and services available to them rather than selecting what they would want in a perfect world. It's hard for a customer to imagine everything that the product could be. It's also rare that an industry will be able to produce collectively products with such infinite variation. Therefore, the manufacturer or supplier typically is forced to narrow the options for the customer.

Lean Thinking helps us get to the customer's true needs.

Value stream, flow, pull, and perfection

The central themes of Lean Thinking are

- value stream
- flow
- pull
- perfection (Womack and Jones, 1996)

Value stream

A **value stream** is a set of actions that produces the products or services needed by the customer. The key is to look at the individual steps in the process that result directly in the provision of the desired services or products. These are considered "value-added" steps.

The **optimized value stream** contains a **minimum** set of activities needed to meet customer needs in a continuous, smooth-flowing process. It has the fewest possible number of non-value-added steps.

Flow

Flow is the progressive achievement of tasks along the **value stream.**

A measurement used to determine flow is **"Takt time."** The term is derived from the German word *taktzeit*, which translates to "clock cycle." Takt time is the pace production needs to meet in order to fill the supply needs of the customer.

Takt time is calculated by dividing the maximum time available to do with work by the time necessary to meet the customer's need. So, for example, if the customer requires the work to be done in one hour and the maximum time available to do the work is one hour, the Takt time is 1 (maximum time available divided by time necessary to meet the customer's need; 1 divided by 1 = 1).

If the customer requires the work to be done in two hours and the maximum time available to do the work is 1 hour, the Takt time is 2 (2 divided by 1 = 2).

If the customer requires the work to be done in 1 hour and the maximum time available to do the work is 2 hours, the Takt time is 0.5 (1 divided by 2 = 0.5).

The Takt time will tell you which processes need to be improved—that is processes with a Takt time greater than 1.

Each separate activity in a process or system is identified and classified as either value-added (to the customer) or non-value-added. The time it takes to perform each task is measured. Non-value-added steps in the process are then eliminated, if possible, or the time it takes to do them is reduced.

| Figure 5.1 | Identifying and reducing non-value-added steps |

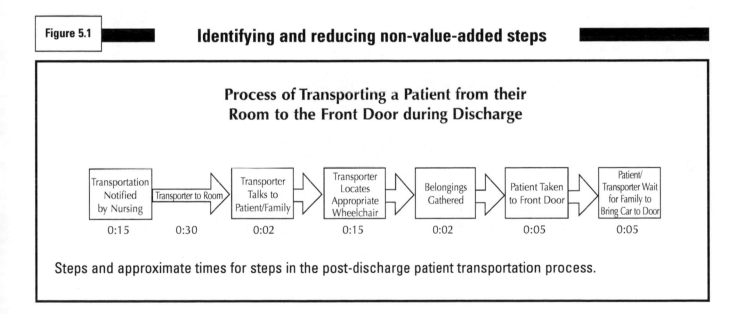

Process of Transporting a Patient from their Room to the Front Door during Discharge

Steps and approximate times for steps in the post-discharge patient transportation process.

Figure 5.2 Identifying and reducing non-value-added steps

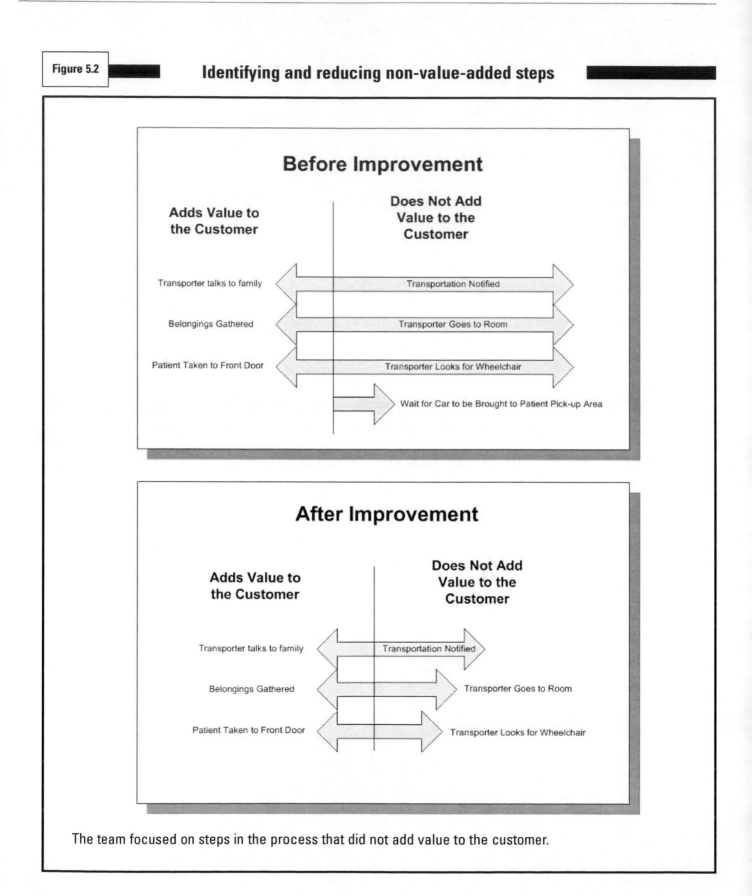

The team focused on steps in the process that did not add value to the customer.

Figure 5.2 shows a very simplified patient transportation process at the time of discharge. Note that the improvement process eliminated one of four non-value-added steps and reduced the time it took for the remaining three.

Pull

Lean's emphasis on **pull** focuses the supply chain on the timing and level of customer demand: It is the need to be able to deliver products to customers as soon as they want them—and not before. Pull provides responsiveness to the true market or customer demand, reduces stockpiling of products, avoids waste due to storage, and reduces the production of material that is no longer desired by the customer.

Perfection

Perfection means just what it sounds like: to continuously strive to improve the product and the production process. The drive toward continuous improvement is constant, and settling on past achievements or success is not acceptable.

KAIZEN BREAKTHROUGH EVENTS IN LEAN THINKING

Kaizen is a Japanese term from two words:

Kai = to break apart, modify, change

Zen = to think about, make good, make better

Kaizen means to break apart and put back together better than before. It is a process to identify and reduce/eliminate waste. It is a process for identifying and implementing standardized work.

The Lean Thinking process

A Lean Thinking application begins when leadership assembles a team dedicated to the rapid delivery of innovation and continuous improvement. Lean Thinking teams are typically cross-functional and work together on the improvement project for three to 10 days, with a scheduled follow-up about 30 days later.

Many organizations use outside consultants to guide them as they get started and teach the themes and techniques of Lean Thinking.

Lean process principles

The Lean Thinking principles are

- eliminate waste
- improve work flow
- optimize inventory
- change the work environment to support elimination of waste
- enhance the customer relationship
- manage time
- manage variation
- design systems to avoid mistakes
- focus on products and services that meet the customer demand

Eliminate waste

There are many types of waste in healthcare. The Lean Thinking term for waste is "muda," the Japanese word for non-value-added activities. There are eight areas of waste:

1. Transportation
2. Motion
3. Waiting
4. Processing
5. Inventory
6. Overproduction
7. Corrections
8. Defects

Figure 5.3 lists some examples of waste in healthcare and their potential causes.

Figure 5.3

Where to look for possible waste (or muda) in the healthcare environment

Muda or Waste	Where to Look in Health Care	Potential Causes
Transportation	• Moving lab samples and specimens from one place to another • Moving patients for tests or treatments • Moving patients for surgery • Moving patients for admission or discharge • Moving papers or documents • Moving equipment	• Poor layout • Lack of coordination of processes • Poor housekeeping • Poor workplace organization • Multiple storage locations
Motion	• Searching for patients • Searching for equipment • Searching for charts or documents • Searching for supplies • Searching for staff or physicians • Poor department layout	• Lack of workplace organization • Poor layout • Inconsistent work methods • Poor designs
Waiting - Delays	• Bed assignments • Admission to the hospital • Admission to the emergency department • Collection of specimens • Performing tests / treatments • Results of testing and treatments • Discharge from the hospital • Test processing	• Inconsistent work methods • Systems or services are not aligned or coordinated • Bottlenecks in supply and demand • Unbalance flow
Processing	• Retesting • Multiple bed moves • Repeat testing and treatments • Unnecessary procedures • Redundant approvals	• Inconsistent systems of communication • Inconsistent work methods • •
Inventory	• Pharmacy Stock • Lab supplies • Material management supplies • Patients in beds • Specimens waiting analysis and release of results	• Inaccurate forecasting • Long change over time • Unreliable equipment • Unbalance flow
Overproduction	• Medication given early to suit staff schedules. • Testing ahead of time to suite the lab schedule	• Lack of communication • Inappropriate reward systems • Focus on keeping busy rather than meeting the customer needs
Correction	• Reviewing charts • Retesting due to error	• Insufficient training • Lack of standardized procedures • Incapable processes
Defects	• Wrong patient, procedure site/side procedure • Testing on the wrong patient • Rework or redraws • Missing information • Patient Falls • Medication Events/errors • Chemical Spills	• Insufficient training • Lack of standardized procedures • Incapable processes

Improving workflow

There is often a mismatch between capacity and demand in healthcare. There are also built-in delays due to lack of coordination.

Improving the workflow of healthcare means identifying and eliminating/reducing bottlenecks, minimizing handoffs, and automation, when possible.

Optimize inventory

Unbalanced inventories (more supplies than required or fewer supplies than required) may be due to

- poor forecasting
- miscommunication
- hoarding

Human beings tend to hoard when they are afraid (often due to bad past experiences) that necessary supplies will not be available when they need them. This is especially true in healthcare, where the supply might be critical to patient care or safety.

Change the work environment to support elimination of waste

Changing the work environment in healthcare is a daunting task. When approaching this challenge, consider that healthcare depends on the rapid flow of information. Providing the information people need, when they need it, makes them more efficient and, therefore, is a potential focus for improvement.

Healthcare involves an overwhelming number of functions, many of which are time sensitive. Simplifying, streamlining, and training staff in these functions is therefore essential.

To be ready for a cultural change where the mantra is to fix it, fix it again, and then fix it again, staff members should be supported with realistic measures, evaluations, and reward systems.

Enhance the customer relationship

Lean Thinking is based on getting customers what they want, when they want it. Focus first on the customer, then apply Lean Thinking processes to make a difference.

Remember, the customer in healthcare is not only the patient: it may also be the physician or other disciplines that support the healthcare system.

Manage time

Waiting is a great waste of time. In many situations, timely care is quality care (such as in the emergency department). Also, customers (patients, physicians, other staff members) become very dissatisfied by unnecessary waits.

Manage variation

Variation is inherent to all processes. The amount of variation, however, can be controlled to give a consistent product or service. Standardization is an important approach to reducing variation. Standardization, in turn, requires operational definitions, protocols, and checklists. But please remember that no matter how standard you make a flawed system, it will yield unacceptable variation: making a bad system more consistent will not necessarily make the outcome (i.e., the product) better.

Design systems to avoid mistakes

Healthcare is loaded with processes that rely on human vigilance to avoid errors or mistakes. It is therefore important to engage in "error-proofing" or designing systems so that simple human diligence is not the only barrier between a process that works and a process that creates an error. Pokayoke is a Japanese term for such mistake-proofing. Examples include

- bar coding for patient identification, lab specimens, medications, etc.
- separating look-alike/sound-alike medications
- specially designed medical gas connections on anesthesia machines
- JCAHO's National Patient Safety Goals

Focus on the product or service that meets the customer demand

Remember to keep the needs of the customer (the VOC, in Six Sigma terms) in mind as you simplify and streamline processes.

Steps in the application of Lean Thinking

Leadership begins by focusing on the goals of the organization and then selects a process for improvement. A team is assembled and begins to receive education regarding the overall Lean Thinking process and expectations for improvement. The team begins by reviewing the existing process, usually using a process-flow map or a flow chart. The team then begins to identify waste and non-value-added activities. During this diagnostic step, the team may use many classic quality improvement tools, such as Pareto diagrams, control charts, and histograms.

The team, along with leadership, creates a vision of the new workflow, specifies an action plan, and measures the performance of the new process. The team participates as the new process is implemented by the involved department(s). The processes is monitored (through periodic checks) through the use of specific process indicators (i.e., lean core measures). These checks are reported to the leaders who sponsored the team.

Lean core measures

The four lean core measures are

1. improving productivity
2. reducing inventory
3. reducing layout
4. reducing lead time

These measures lead to higher quality—that is, less waste, lower costs, and improved customer satisfaction. Patient satisfaction can be damaged when defects occur, such as an error in testing or treatment; when there is a delay in service; when an item that is needed by the patient, such as a lab result is lost. Applying Lean Thinking to the reduction of such events adds to patient satisfaction. The cost of poor quality can be addressed with the reduction of waste and increased efficiency.

Specific tools of Lean Thinking

Tool: Workplace organization techniques, or the discipline of 5-S

The concept of 5-S is based on the Japanese approach to an organized environment, as follows:

- Organization (**seiri**)—Keeping on hand only what is needed for the process
- Orderliness (**seiton**)—A place for everything and everything in its place for immediate use
- Cleanliness (**seiso**)—Keep the workplace clean, spotless, and shining
- Standardized cleanup (**seiketsu**)—It creates a condition for repeating the successes in the future
- Discipline (**shitsuke**)—Through the strength of personal will and self-esteem, make a habit of maintaining the established procedures everyday

The goal is to create a workplace that supports the new process and that can keep the new process in motion.

Tool: Standardized operations

Standardized operations are used to set guidelines for how each process should be performed. This improves efficiency and consistency in performance and outcomes. The focus is to assist the employee. Standardized operations document each step in the process. They can, and usually do, document the duration or time of each step. This provides a graphic depiction of movements and identifies workloads.

Tool: Standardize process for continuous flow

Work is organized with no

- waiting or walking
- looking for supplies, equipment, or information

The physical layout supports efficiency of the workflow. When using Lean Thinking, people often identify waste with re-work or with delays that result because the process is poorly defined and the worker is subjected to constant changes in the environment.

Tool: Takt time

As explained in the beginning of this section, the Takt time is the actual time it takes to produce products or services relative to the needs of the customers.

Other QI tools commonly used in Lean Thinking

- Simple flow charts and process mapping (to identify non-value- and value-added steps to a process)

- Time-function mapping (showing the relationship of time elapsed and time expected to perform the various steps of a process or time to produce one unit, product, or service)

- Relationship mapping (to show how the various steps of a process are organized)

- Pareto chart (ranked data to show the contribution of each measured item)

- Control charts (to distinguish between common cause and special cause variation)

- Cause-and-effect charts or "Ishikawa" diagrams (to identify factors that contribute to a process)

- Failure modes and effects analysis (FMEA) (to identify and prioritize the "failure modes" of a process)

- Fault tree analysis (to help identify the root cause of a potential failure).

LEAN THINKING RESOURCES

James Womack and Daniel Jones, *Lean Thinking: Banish Waste and Create Wealth in Your Corporation, 2nd Edition*.

James Womack and Daniel Jones, *The Machine that Changed the World*.

Ricki Stajer, *Applying Principles of Lean Process Improvement* (VHA, Inc., April 18, 2002 presentation).

Takt Time Efficiency Displays, www.vorne.com.

www.leanhealthcare.com – Gemba Research.

LEAN THINKING CASE STUDY: FINDING THE WHEELCHAIR

One hospital used Lean Thinking tools to great effect by solving delays in the transportation of discharged patients. A two-hour wait was not uncommon between the time transportation was requested and the time the patient had left the room.

Leadership identified this as a priority for improvement because of the "upstream" impacts of this "downstream" delay. Excessive delays in discharge (due, in part, to delays in transportation) meant delays in making the bed available for the next admission. This meant that inpatients were kept in the emergency department, filling up the hallways to the point that new patients brought in by paramedics had to be kept in the paramedic ambulance that brought them. The ambulance was therefore not available for the next run. There were actually times in this community when all available paramedic ambulances were parked outside this hospital's emergency department and were therefore not available to respond to the next 911 call.

Like Six Sigma, Lean Thinking must connect with the institution's financial bottom line. The connection in this case was easy: The cost of delayed transports added to the costs of missed admissions and extended lengths of stay.

The quality and safety impacts of this issue were likewise self-evident.

Creating the team

Like all good quality projects, the Lean Thinking improvement team included the folks actually doing the work (transporters), other staff involved in the discharge process (nurses, ward clerks, etc.), and the nursing director (who was also the leadership sponsor).

Working the problem

Figure 5.2 illustrates a simplified flow chart of the discharge transportation process and a sample of how value-added and non-value-added steps were identified. This was the first part of the team's work (facilitated by an external consultant).

Reducing the time for "finding the wheelchair"

Lean Thinking tools are quite powerful when applied to the right problem. The way in which this team found a key flaw in the transportation process illustrates this point nicely.

CASE STUDY	LEAN THINKING CASE STUDY: FINDING THE WHEELCHAIR (CONT.)

Remember, an important part of Lean Thinking improvement processes is the reduction of the time it takes to perform non-value-added steps. It is therefore necessary that you know the current time it takes to do each step in the process.

The time it takes a transporter to find a wheelchair is definitely NOT a valuable expense of time from the patient's point of view. Therefore, the team set out to measure how long it really took to perform this step. Two members of the team were assigned to follow each transporter through daily tasks. In Lean Thinking, these types of observations a very structured and focused:

- One person followed the transporter to list each successive activity performed
- The second person noted the time it took to perform each task

The team was amazed when they gathered at the end of the day to analyze their findings. Here is one set of observations:

- Transporter assigned to take John Doe from room 101 to the front door for discharge
- Travel to room 101 (0:02)
- Interaction with patient and family (0:01)
- Travel to elevator lobby of first floor to find available wheelchair (unsuccessful) (0:01)
- Travel to elevator lobby of second floor to find available wheelchair (successful) (0:01)
- Travel to room 101 with wheelchair (0:02)
- Attempt to transfer patient to wheelchair (unsuccessful: wheelchair too small) (0:05)
- Return wheelchair to elevator lobby (0:01)
- Travel to elevator lobby of first floor to find available "big boy" wheelchair (unsuccessful) (0:01)
- Respond to page from supervisor (0.02)
- Travel to elevator lobby of second floor to find available "big boy" wheelchair (unsuccessful) (0:02)
- Travel to elevator lobby of third floor to find available "big boy" wheelchair (unsuccessful) (0:01)

LEAN THINKING CASE STUDY:
FINDING THE WHEELCHAIR (CONT.)

- Travel to elevator lobby of fourth floor to find available "big boy" wheelchair (unsuccessful) (0:02)
- Travel to elevator lobby of fifth floor to find available "big boy" wheelchair (SUCCESS!!) (0:01)
- Travel to room 101 with wheelchair (0:02)
- Transfer patient (0:03)
- Respond to page from supervisor (0.02)
- Travel to front door (0:02)
- Wait for car to be pulled around (0:05)
- Transfer patient to car (0:05)
- Return wheelchair to elevator lobby (0:01)
- Transporter available for next assignment

(Total time: approximately 40 minutes. During that 40 minutes, five other unmet requests for transportation were received.)

You probably see the point. The hospital standardized where wheelchairs were kept and bought two more oversized models. More importantly, the Lean Thinking approach and tools made a significant difference to the patient discharge transportation process. The approach also positively impacted a number of other issues at this and other institutions.

CHAPTER SIX

BALANCED SCORECARD

BALANCED SCORECARD

ELEVATOR DESCRIPTION OF BALANCED SCORECARD

Quick: You have a two-floor ride in an elevator with your CEO and medical director and they want to know about Balanced Scorecard.

A Balanced Scorecard is a method to organize, communicate, and measure performance on the most important aspects of the organization based on its business plan and strategic goals.

Wait a minute! We already have a scorecard: It's called a financial statement. Managers up and down the organization already are held accountable for how they perform compared to budget. Why would we need or want something other than that?

- A financial report is a "lagging" report: that is, it doesn't tell you where you're going, it tells you where you've been. Although we'll always be held accountable for the financial bottom line, it is essential to develop "predictive" or concurrent measures as well to see whether you're on course.

- It's hard to steer a car down the highway by only looking in the rearview mirror.

To use Balanced Scorecards effectively develop a system of scorecards that addresses performance at all levels: the organizational level, the divisional level, and the unit or service level.

Balanced Scorecards do the following:

- Align vision and mission with customer requirements and daily work

- Manage and evaluate business strategies
- Monitor operational efficiency improvements
- Communicate progress to all employees

Balanced Scorecards translate the corporate vision into actionable activities for all departments and units. This method provides a common language to say what needs to be done in an organization and what the targets or goals are. Balanced Scorecards also provide feedback regarding current performance in relation to those targets or goals.

Figure 6.1

Vision/Mission

Area	Strategic goals	Actions or strategies
Finance	• OB hospital days will be X • The monthly budget will be within X% of goal	• Monitor payroll and non-payroll costs • Monitor overtimes and incidental costs
Service	• Increase OB satisfaction scores to X% • Review Federal Emergency Medical Treatment and Active Labor Act (EMTALA)	• Improve pain management during labor • Improve information given to new mothers regarding self care and baby care • Improve the discharge process • Review processes to support appropriate EMTALA requirements
Clinical quality	• Improve pain management during labor • Improve information given to new mothers regarding self care and baby care • Conduct preoperative or invasive procedure briefings	• Pain assessment skills for nurses • Pain management with anesthesia • Develop new mother and baby educational process
Human Resources	• Reduce turnover rate for first- year nurses • Reduce turnover rate for nurses employed more than one year • Reduce vacancy rate	• Assess needs of new nurses • Preceptor program for new nurses • Employ patient safety briefings to improve teamwork • Assess needs of nurses employed more than one year • Hire the best nurses available and retain them
Community / Corporate Citizen	• Reduce incidence in the community of abandoned babies	• Develop campaign to work with at-risk groups regarding a "Do Not Abandon Your Baby" program

What do we mean when we say a scorecard is "balanced"? We mean that it looks at performance from a number of different perspectives. Scorecards typically become balanced when they examine the following four domains:

1. Financial performance
2. Customer opinions and perspective
3. Internal operational performance
4. Employee learning and growth

Figure 6.2	**Four domains addressed by Balanced Scorecards**

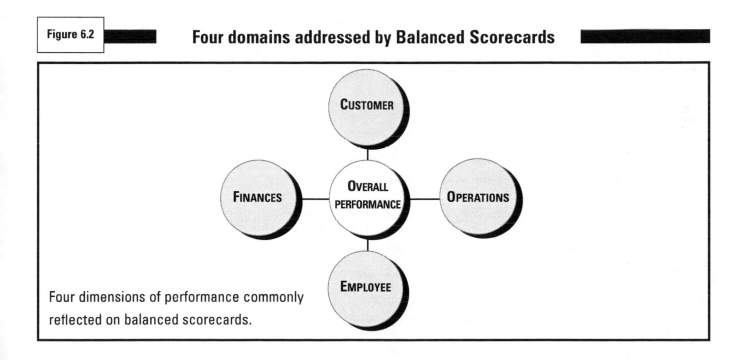

Four dimensions of performance commonly reflected on balanced scorecards.

In order to take the right action at the right time, know the specific performance of these key organizational domains and how the domains are interrelated. Selecting the right measures is fundamental to managing performance effectively.

Just think about how a baseball team measures performance. After each game, the final score is posted along with statistics for each player: batting average, number of strike outs, runs batted in, earned run average, etc. These and other numbers are examined as averages over the entire season and in terms of recent performance. These two perspectives give the manager the necessary information to adjust player line-up for the next game.

A Balanced Scorecard with the right performance measures should do the same for hospital leadership: it provides average and trending information so leadership may make necessary adjustments or provide reinforcement of a job well done.

There are two phases in developing such a Balanced Scorecard: building and implementing.

Building a scorecard

In preparation for building a scorecard, leadership must commit to the process and to the use of the scorecard product. Neglecting this step can mean that leadership doesn't use this management tool, which is the problem that most often causes Balanced Scorecards to fail. There are many outside consultants available to assist the organization through this process, and using one can help spur feelings of urgency and need for follow-though.

Once leadership commitment is secured, a group of senior leaders, quality personnel, and staff to collect the data needs to be assembled. This group is responsible for overseeing the Balanced Scorecard development process. It develops a communication plan regarding how this management tool is to be used and what it means for managers and staff.

Remember that using a Balanced Scorecard probably means a cultural change is necessary for the organization. It means that the most important strategic and operational goals will be measured and displayed, and that actions will be developed in the event that there are gaps in performance.

Although approaches vary slightly, a six-step Balanced Scorecard approach is common.

During each step, the activities are applied to each of the four areas Balanced Scorecards address: financial, customer, internal business process, and learning and growth. This process turns your vision into initiatives to improve the organization.

Step 1—Assessment

The first step is to assess the organization's beliefs, values, market opportunities, competition, and financial position, as well as the customer's needs. Most organizations complete this step so they have a business plan to communicate to stakeholders and other financially interested parties. A SWOT (strengths, weaknesses, opportunities, and threats) analysis often is conducted in this step. Targeted stakeholders that are essential to the business are identified, as are gaps in performance, from the perspective of each external stakeholder.

Step 2—Strategy

This step is dictated by the business strategy, which should be guided by what will make the organization most successful. Business strategies usually focus on areas such as growing, meeting business/regulatory requirements, and providing services.

Step 3—Objectives

Once business strategies are selected, break them into smaller "bite-sized" pieces. Doing so transforms them into tangible business or strategic objectives, which are goals that will lead the organization to a higher level of performance.

Step 4—Strategic map

Each objective or goal is then "mapped" to the appropriate scorecard "domain" (financial, customer, operations, and learning and growth).

If the objective is to increase nurse retention, then it is linked to learning and growth of the organization. Increased nurse retention is, in turn, linked to customer satisfaction due to the development of the retained nurses to provide customer service and expertise.

| Figure 6.3 | **Strategic cycle or map** | |

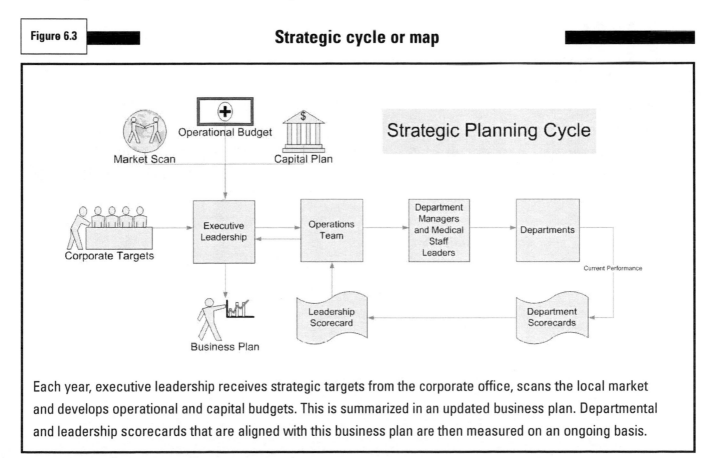

Each year, executive leadership receives strategic targets from the corporate office, scans the local market and develops operational and capital budgets. This is summarized in an updated business plan. Departmental and leadership scorecards that are aligned with this business plan are then measured on an ongoing basis.

Step 5—Performance measures

Specific performance measures are then developed. Using a strategic map, key objectives are selected and the most appropriate and powerful indicator available is used to measure progression toward that indicator.

• Selecting the right measure

Because the number of measures will be small, their quality must be high. They must be the best, most reliable indicators focused on exactly the right subject. It is natural and appropriate to start with a review of existing measures, but it is often necessary to modify them or develop new ones to measure a specific issue accurately, consistently, and readily.

• Narrowing the focus

Although it may be tempting to look at a lot of measures, too many can become overwhelming and cause the scorecard to fail (a common problem). But how many measures are too many? This is an ongoing balancing act. There must be enough measures to give an overall picture of performance, but the number of indicators must not overwhelm the folks responsible for their collection, analysis, and display.

Also, the oversight group must be able to focus on the right aspects. Ideally, all measures would be displayed on a **single page.**

Step 6—Initiatives

Initiatives are then funded and staffed to improve performance (when indicated). Desired outcomes are communicated to the teams working on the initiatives. This step does not direct the organization regarding specific quality improvement methodology tools to be used, so organizations will select Six Sigma, Lean Thinking, or other methods described in this book.

The power of a scorecard to align efforts

Developing a Balanced Scorecard using this method is a powerful way to align improvement efforts. Prior to the alignment of the strategy, objective, and initiative, everyone works based only on their own knowledge of what is important to the organization—an incomplete picture at best.

After the key objectives of the organization are clarified through the Balanced Scorecard, however, improvement efforts can be better prioritized and aligned.

Figure 6.4

Alignment of improvement activities
before the Balanced Scorecard

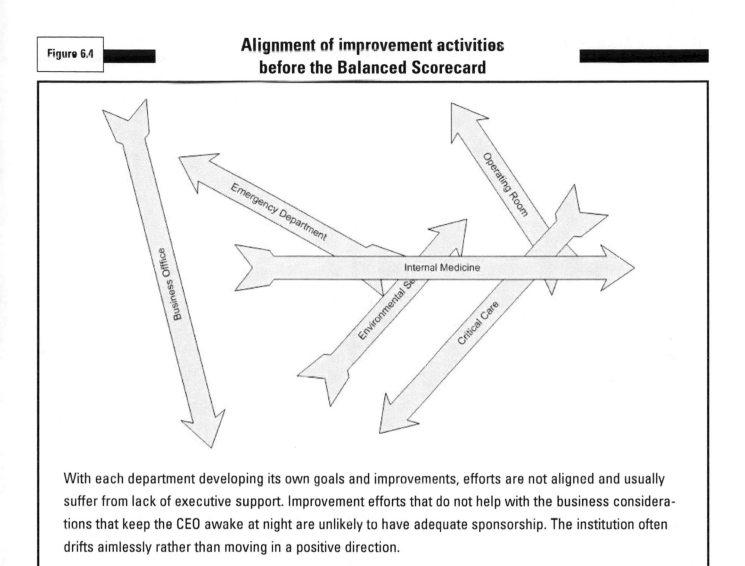

With each department developing its own goals and improvements, efforts are not aligned and usually suffer from lack of executive support. Improvement efforts that do not help with the business considerations that keep the CEO awake at night are unlikely to have adequate sponsorship. The institution often drifts aimlessly rather than moving in a positive direction.

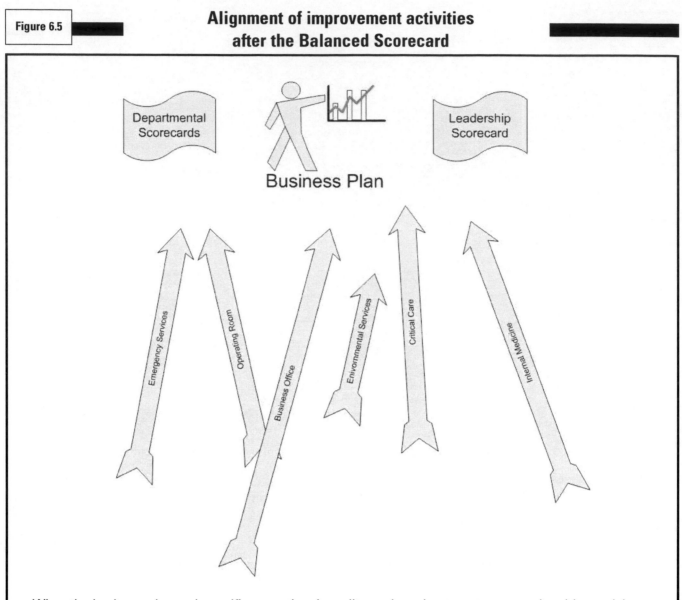

Figure 6.5

Alignment of improvement activities after the Balanced Scorecard

When the business plan and specific operational, quality, and service targets are used to drive activities, performance improvement efforts align and the institution moves forward.

Scorecard format

Balanced Scorecards are displayed in various formats. They may focus on strategic maps, performance measures, new initiatives, or outcomes. Most organizations use a performance measures focus to get a real-time sense of success, but using an initiative focus is also useful, as it lets leadership know how improvement is applied.

Some organizations install computer software that displays real-time scorecards. For example, hotel chains typically have an executive information system that displays the occupancy rate (and other measures) across the system. The executive can, with the touch of a button, drill down through the various levels to show divisional, regional, or individual hotel performance.

A few hospitals and healthcare systems have gone a short distance down this road. For example, some hospitals have executive flow management computer scorecards that show available beds, number of admissions waiting in the ED, etc. However, overall healthcare performance scorecards are much more difficult to automate. Most of us are still struggling to extract information manually from the medical record to calculate some measures.

Organizations illustrate their performance in many ways. Some use a spider diagram (see Figure 6.7) showing gaps between current performance and targets. Some use a picture that looks like a gas gauge with the needle on full (meeting the target) or empty (not meeting the target). A report card format is common with a grade (score) in colors (i.e., green for meeting target, yellow for caution or close to meeting the target, and red for not meeting the target. Charts and graphs are frequently used with a comment on the target and the current performance. Imagine ways to communicate your progress to your organization.

The intent is to get everyone in the organization knowledgeable regarding the most important things to the success of the organization. When implemented, leadership and staff should be able to identify what their contribution is to the organization's success.

Figure 6.6	Balanced Scorecard example

STRATEGIC GOALS SCORECARD –PERINATAL SERVICES

Key: ☺ = Meets or Exceeds Target; ☺ = Within 5% of target; ☹ = Greater than 5% adverse to target / target not met; ↑ = Significant improvement since previous reporting period.

	☺	☺	☹			☺	☺	☹
Affordability					**Clinical Quality**			
Obstetrical Hospital Days will be 2.7 or less	☺				Patients will report satisfaction with labor pain management in the 75th percentile			☹
Financial performance will be within 2% of target		☺						
Personalized Care					90% of postpartum mothers will demonstrate good understanding of well baby care prior to discharge.			☹
Access								
External review of EMALA compliance will demonstrate no barriers to care	☺				There will be no complications related to vaginal births after cesarean section (VBAC).	☺		
Patient Perception					**Regulatory Compliance**			
Patient satisfaction with OB services will be in the 75 percentile		☺			No action plan targets will be missed for the current periodic performance review.		☺	
The median time from discharge order to transport will be less than 20 minutes	☺↑				**People**			
					Turnover rate will be less than 1%	☺		
Safety Experience					RN Vacancy Rate will be less than 1%		☺	
The pre-procedure pause will be conducted 100% of the time			☹		**Community Service**			
					All community service goals will be met.		☺	

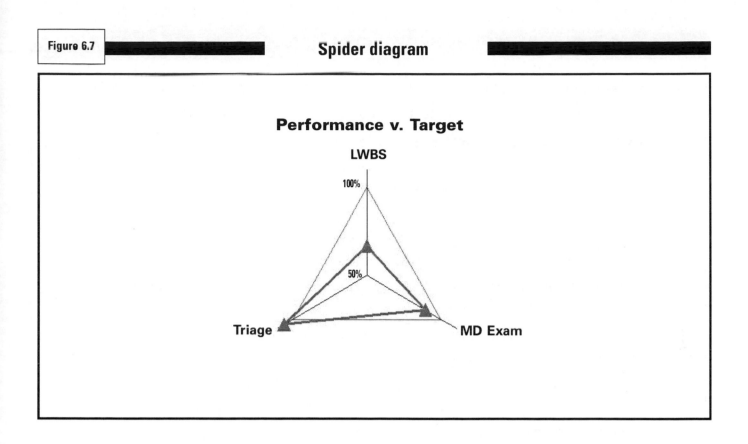

Figure 6.7   **Spider diagram**

Performance v. Target

Implementation

A Balanced Scorecard creates a system of accountability and responsibility for the strategic goals of the organization. Its successful implementation depends on communication.

Quality professionals cannot be the sole keepers of Balanced Scorecards—leadership has to show they are going to use the information from the performance measures. In addition, the team that was brought together to work on the Balanced Scorecard must develop the communication plan.

Measures and targets are commonly displayed and initiatives or actions are evaluated to determine whether they are improving the organization. The power of using the Balanced Scorecard tool is that goals are visible to leadership, managers, and staff. It leaves no room for misinterpretation of what is considered important or how well the organization is performing. Ideally all improvement efforts (resources) would be spent on projects that will positively impact one or more scorecard measures.

IMPLEMENTATION QUESTIONS

The following questions should be addressed before you begin to implement a Balanced Scorecard. The questions need to be answered by the team assembled to construct the Balanced Scorecard and by leadership.

- Who will use the Balanced Scorecard? (Will it be senior leaders, managers, or staff?)
- How will the Balanced Scorecard be used? (In monthly meetings, to create management and staff accountability?)
- How will the Balanced Scorecard be made available? (Through meetings, postings, mailers, newsletters, or company intranet sites?)
- How will the Balanced Scorecards be developed? (With senior leaders, management, staff, or focus groups?)
- How will data be collected and incorporated into the Balanced Scorecard?
- Who will collect data and incorporate it into the Balanced Scorecard?
- How often will data be collected and displayed?
- How will managers be trained to use the Balanced Scorecard?
- Will the Balanced Scorecard results be tied to performance incentives for leadership, management, and staff?

Refreshing the Balanced Scorecard

The indicators in a Balanced Scorecard should be reviewed and revised if necessary, with each new business cycle. The Balanced Scorecard can also be amended mid-cycle if new opportunities are identified.

BALANCED SCORECARD RESOURCES

Arthur M. Schneiderman, "Why Balanced Scorecards Fail!", *Journal of Strategic Performance Measurement,* (January 1999 Special Edition).

Howard Rohm, "A Balancing Act" *Perform,* Vol 2 Issue 2

Kaplan and Nolan, *The Balanced Scorecard by* (Harvard Business School Press).

CASE STUDY	BALANCED SCORECARD EXAMPLE: MANAGING PATIENT FLOW

We are not the only people who believe in the power of a Balanced Scorecard for healthcare. The Joint Commission on Accreditation of Healthcare Organizations (JCAHO), when it adopted standard LD.3.15 (effective January 1, 2005), essentially mandated that accredited hospitals develop a Balanced Scorecard to address patient flow. Here's how one organization designed its patient flow scorecard:

Leadership began by gathering a team, including

- the chief operating officer
- the nursing manager of the emergency department
- the physician leader (chief) of emergency medicine
- the physician chair of the utilization management (resource management) committee
- the director of quality
- the chief financial officer
- the nurse executive
- the director of case management
- a data analyst

The team identified key objectives related to

a. supply of patient bed space
b. efficiency of patient care and treatment areas
c. safety of patient care and treatment areas
d. support service processes that impact patient flow

Existing indicators were reviewed and a list of candidate scorecard measures was developed. The list included far more measures than they could possibly collect, display, and analyze in a meaningful way. Ultimately, the list was whittled down to a precious few.

CASE STUDY	BALANCED SCORECARD EXAMPLE: MANAGING PATIENT FLOW (CONT.)

Figure 4.5 — **Patient flow scorecard**

Indicator	Nov '03	Dec'03	Jan '04	Feb '04	Mar '04	Apr '04	Target	12-Month Rolling Average	☺☺☹
Volumes									
Number of ED Visits	3325	3615	3725	3200	3013	3050	-	3215	
Inpatient Occupancy	91.0%	92.5%	92.0%	90.5%	87.0%	88.0%			
Percentage of Admission	15.6%	16.7%	17.1%	16.4%	14.5%	15.8%	-	15.8%	
Emergency Department Impact									
Left Without Being Seen	6.5%	5.0%	5.5%	6.0%	4.4%	3.9%	4%	5.5%	☹
Percent of Patients Highly Satisfied with ED Care		75%			74%		90%	75%	☹
Percent Urgent Patients Seen by Provider within 1 Hour	60%	55%	65%	75%	86%	83%	80%	81%	☺
Average LOS: Admitted Patients	6.1	6.2	6.5		5.85	5.9	-	6.1	
Percent of Admitted Patients Placed in Inpatient Bed Within 2 Hours of Admitting Order	58%	35%	42%	68%	75%	78%	80%	62%	☹
% Door to Therapy in 30 Min	91%		89%		93%		90%	92%	☺
% Agency Use	3%	8%	14%	9%	8%	2%	4%	5%	☹
Actual Costs to Target	5%	7%	8%	-1%	-3%	-2%	0%	2%	☹
Inpatient Flow									
Number of Boarder-Hours in the Emergency Department	625	780	725	450	376	354	150	514	☹
Number of Boarder-Hours in the Post Anesthesia Recovery Unit	103	98	111	35	25	10	50	45	☺
Percent of Hours on Paramedic Diversion	33%	34%	43%	15%	17%	13%	-	18%	
Average Time of Day for Discharge Order	13:20	13:25	14:30	14:10	13:53	12:55	13:00	13:50	☹
Percent of Patients Discharged Within 2 Hours of Discharge Order	65%	76%	54%	67%	73%	69%	0.9	60%	☹
Patient Safety									
Events Occurring to Boarded Inpatients (See Detailed Listing)	None	2	None	3	None				
Events Occurring to Patients in Temporary Bed Spaces (See Detailed Listing)	1	None	None	None	1				

Leadership can use this scorecard as it monitors improvements to patient flow.

Within a few months of implementation, performance began to improve. Some improvements may have been related to the "Hawthorne effect" (i.e., performance begins to improve merely because it is being measured). The larger impact, however, was due to the focusing of improvement activities. All parties were held accountable for performance related to these indicators. (*Note:* The scorecard displayed in Figure 4.5 was leadership's overall scorecard. There were also department-level scorecards aligned with the leadership version.) This made it easy for efforts to be focused and, therefore, more effective.

CHAPTER SEVEN

ISO 9000

ISO 9000

Quick: You have a two-floor ride in an elevator with your CEO and medical director and they want to know about ISO 9000.

The ISO 9000 standards provide a comprehensive operational framework intended to increase quality, reliability, and efficiency by focusing on the structural details of an organization's internal quality improvement process.

Common terms:

- **ISO:** the International Organization for Standardization
- **ISO 9000:** A series of standards (including ISO 9001:2000, ISO 9002, etc.) focused on a company's quality management system.
- **ISO 9000 Registration:** Evidence of compliance with the ISO 9000 standards. Registration is not awarded by ISO—it may be obtained through many different ISO consulting groups.

The International Organization for Standardization is an agency that has been developing voluntary standards since 1947. The mission of ISO is to promote the worldwide standardization of business processes to facilitate the international exchange of goods and services, and to develop cooperation in the areas of intellectual, scientific, technological, and economic activity.

The ISO 9000 standards offer a rigorous model for documenting an organization's quality improvement process. An organization's adherence to the ISO standards is evidence that it consistently ensures and improves the quality and efficiency of its products and services. According to ISO, compliance with its standards yields improved service, fewer adverse events, and lower costs. And because the ISO 9000 standards apply to a company's quality management system, not to its products, it can be applied to virtually any industry.

The ISO publishes several standards sets, and the ISO 9000 series is aimed at a company's quality management system. Within this series, the ISO 9001:2000 standard is best suited to most healthcare organizations.

ISO 9000 standards should be applied during the contracting process to increase customer confidence in the supplier's systems.

Although the standards prescribe what activities or tasks need to be done, they do not tell you how to accomplish them. The three basic requirements of ISO 9000 are as follows:

- Processes that impact quality are documented
- Records are maintained and data are captured to measure the quality of the goods or services produced
- Operational processes produce consistent quality

Please don't confuse meeting the ISO standards with adhering to the Joint Commission on Accreditation of Healthcare Organizations (JCAHO) or similar standards; the ISO certification process is much more focused and rigorous. However, the ISO standards are more general than JCAHO's very prescriptive requirements.

JCAHO	ISO 9000
Detailed standards	General standards
Specific to the type of healthcare organization	General applicability to various industries
Adherence attested to by JCAHO directly	Adherence attested to by independent contractor
Survey process hit or miss	Very thorough registration process

This standards-based approach to improvement stems from the following logic:

- To consistently meet the customers' specifications, you must eliminate variation in the production process.
- To eliminate variation in the production process, you must make sure that all employees are doing the same thing.
- To make sure employees are following the same process, it must be documented and consistently implemented.
- To make sure the process yields a good product, it must be improved continuously.

ISO 9000 series

The ISO 9000 *quality of system standards* provides a selection of standard sets aimed at various industry types. All of the 9000 standards are aimed at achieving customer satisfaction by meeting their specifications. They also focus on meeting external regulatory requirements and continuous improvement.

The following list gives the titles of the various ISO 9000 standards, which indicate their area of focus:

- **ISO 9000:** *Quality Management and Quality Assurance Standards*. This is the umbrella standard (over ISO 9001, 9002, etc.), and it guides you in determining which subset is right for your organization.
- **ISO 9001:** *Quality Systems–Model for Quality Assurance in Design, Development, Production and Services*. This is the most comprehensive of the 9000 series and applies to all aspects of the production process.
- **ISO 9002:** *Quality Systems–Model for Quality Assurance in Production*.
- **ISO 9003:** *Quality Systems–Model for Quality Assurance in Final Inspection and Testing*.
- **ISO 9004:** *Quality Management and Quality Systems Elements*. This standard provides guidelines for implementing of a quality system and for interpreting standards.

The main sections of the ISO 9001:2000 are as follows:

- **Quality management system**—a collection of processes, documents, resources, and monitoring systems that direct the work of the organization
- **Management responsibility**—requires involvement and commitment of the organization's leaders
- **Resource management**—requires the people, equipment, tools, and materials needed to build the quality management system, improve effectiveness, and meet customer requirements

- **Product realization**—the work an organization does to develop, produce, and deliver products or services (also known as a quality plan)
- **Measurement, analysis, and improvement**—ensure that the product or service is meeting requirements defined though inspection, testing, measurement, analysis, and, when needed, improvement

Healthcare and ISO 9001:2000

There is a general belief that applying ISO 9001:2000 to healthcare will bring benefits. However, there is an "industry-to-healthcare" translation barrier to overcome:

1. The language of healthcare is different than the language of manufacturing and other industries. ISO refers to the *customer*; healthcare refers to the *patient*. ISO speaks of *product* or *service nonconformity*; healthcare instead talks about *incidents or adverse occurrences*.

2. Unlike most other large industries, healthcare is a craft practiced differently by different artisans (e.g., physicians).

3. The number and complexity of the various interactive healthcare systems is mind-boggling: from medication management to operative procedures to supply management to hotel services to nursing practice to ancillary testing to—you get the idea.

Figure 7.1	**Healthcare organizations using ISO**

There are a few hospitals in the United States that have become ISO 9001:2000 certified or registered. American Legion Hospital in Crowley, LA, is believed to have been the first in North America, registered under ISO 9002. Laboratories are more commonly ISO certified or registered than are hospitals.

There are also some small physician-based practices that have become ISO certified or registered. It has been reported that there are only about 100 in North America and more than 400 in Europe.

In addition, many of the companies that provide equipment and supplies to hospitals are ISO registered, as are many of the employers in the communities hospitals serve.

Because of these and other issues, documenting and implementing these processes and the quality improvement practices that apply to them is not simple—but it can be very worthwhile.

ISO 9000's quality model

ISO 9001:2000 requires the institution to use some version of the Shewhart Cycle (described in Chapter 1) to ensure continuous improvement. Various versions of the PDCA (Plan, Do, Check, Act) approach will work. For example, one could easily fit the Six Sigma DMAIC model into the PDCA paradigm.

A systems example of the PDCA application could be seen as follows:

- Plan—Customer requirements, individual patient events, the healthcare market demands by payer, and regulatory agencies
- Do—Diagnosis, patient plan of care, patient treatment, information flow, resource planning, and provision
- Check—Patient satisfaction, best practices, measure and analyze
- Act—Policy and objectives review, strategic information

PDCA is a common problem-solving cycle used by many organizations seeking improvement. In ISO, the improvement process is implemented and documented using this framework.

Becoming "ISO registered"

There are multiple ways in which an organization can become ISO registered. A common course of action includes the following steps:

- *Leadership decides to become* ISO *registered*—leadership commitment is essential to a successful application.
- *Purchase the standard* and become familiar with its requirements.
- *Review support literature and software*—there are many tools that have been created by consultants to aid the organization through the ISO process.
- *Assemble a team*—establish responsibilities for the implementation process with the involvement of senior leadership.
- *Consider training*—there are many courses available to aid the organization.
- *Review potential consultants*—using a consultant in the process can be very helpful, can reduce rework, and can speed up the process.
- *Implement the quality management system*—gap analysis, policies, and procedures must be documented and staff must be trained to use them.

- *Review management system effectiveness*—collect data and review the system; this is one of the final stages of implementation. A continual improvement strategy is to check that your system is both working effectively and conforming to the requirements of ISO 9001:2000.
- *Choose a registrar*—a third party who assesses the effectiveness of the quality management system and will issue a certificate if it meets the standards' requirements.
- *Gain registration*—the key step in the process is a registration assessment, at which time the quality management system is assessed.

ISO certification and registration

First, a definition of terms:

Certification: An independent firm certifies that you meet the ISO standards.
Registration: After confirming that you meet the ISO standards, an independent firm enters you into their registry of ISO-certified organizations.

In practice, these terms are used interchangeably. Certification/registration is the most common way to demonstrate compliance with ISO standards. However, some organizations follow the ISO standards without seeking formal registration; they realize the benefits of a solid quality process without the need to go though initial and ongoing reviews by an external consulting group.

To become certified, an independent approved third-party registrar must audit the company to assess whether it conforms to the standard. There is an off-site review of the manual that describes the quality process and all of the supporting documents. This review is followed by an on-site review of the quality system. If the company is found to be in conformance with the quality system standards, the company is then recommended for ISO registration. Registration means that the auditing body records the certification in its register. Annual audits by both independent and in-house personnel ensure continued compliance with the standard.

Choosing a registrar must be done carefully. The group must be able to demonstrate understanding of and experience with your business. Remember, there is a wide range of industries seeking ISO registration.

Some healthcare organizations have reported increased business due to ISO registration or even due to acknowledging that they follow the ISO standards. Why? Because ISO speaks in a language the rest of the business world understands. Whereas the banker on the board of trustees or the manufacturer selecting a health plan for his employees understands ISO registration, they would be hard-pressed to explain the benefit of JCAHO accreditation.

Results of the ISO 9000 investment

The following results have been reported by institutions that follow the ISO standards:

- Market share has increased due to recognition of the ISO achievement
- Non-value-added activities, such as repair or rework, have been reduced or eliminated
- Employees are empowered to stop work when they believe the work is not correct
- Each employee has the right and is encouraged to report quality problems
- Customer satisfaction with the product or service has increased

In summary, using an organized framework such as ISO 9000 to assess the business processes, to make concerted efforts to manage those processes, and to measure the processes and outcomes provides a sound approach to improvement.

ISO RESOURCES

"A Guide for the Adoption of ISO 9001:2000 in Healthcare," *www.bsonline.techindex.co.uk.*

"American National Standard," American Society for Quality Control, WI.

Jeanne Ketola and Kathy Roberts, *ISO 9000:2000 In a Nutshell, Second Edition.*

International Standard ISO 9002, *www.iso.org.*

ISO 9000 guidelines for health care sector, ISO Management Systems (December 2001).

Quality Council of India, Check up on the use of IWA 1 and ISO 9001:2000 in Health Services. *www.qcin.org/html/nqc/nqc_news7.htm.*

"Successful ISO 9000:2000 Implementation Made Easy," *www.bsiamericas.com.*

Welcome to ISO easy! *www.isoeasy.org*

"What is ISO 9001:2000?" BSI Management Systems.

CHAPTER EIGHT

THE MALCOLM BALDRIGE NATIONAL QUALITY AWARD

CHAPTER EIGHT

THE MALCOLM BALDRIGE NATIONAL QUALITY AWARD

ELEVATOR DESCRIPTION OF BALDRIGE

Quick: You have a two-floor ride in an elevator with your CEO and medical director and they want to know about the Malcolm Baldrige National Quality Award.

The Malcolm Baldrige National Quality Award is non-prescriptive, criteria-based frame-work that guides organizations to improve their products and services, their customers' satisfaction, and their financial bottom line by achieving world-class performance.

The Malcolm Baldrige National Quality Award (MBNQA) is given by the President of the United States to organizations that are judged to be outstanding in seven areas:

1. Leadership
2. Strategic planning
3. Customer and market focus
4. Information and analysis
5. Human resource focus
6. Process management
7. Business results

Vetting for this annual award takes more than 1,000 hours by various examiners.

The MBNQA is given to the following industries:

- Manufacturing (small and large)
- Service (small and large)
- Healthcare
- Education

The MBNQA is awarded annually; however, it is withheld if none of the applicants score above the minimum threshold.

The History of the MBNQA

Congress started the MBNQA in 1987 as a standard of excellence that would help organizations achieve world-class quality and performance. It was intended to raise awareness of the importance of quality and performance for U.S. companies that were losing market share to foreign interests.

Malcolm Baldrige was the Secretary of Commerce from 1981 until his accidental death in 1987. He was a proponent of helping U.S. business become world-class and he helped draft the early versions of the award. Congress named the award in his honor.

The Baldrige criteria are written to provide a robust framework for an organization to hold itself accountable. The criteria do not tell the organization how to achieve them. Rather, the intent is to enhance competitiveness by focusing on delivering improving value to customers and improving overall organizational performance.

Its original roots were in Total Quality Management (TQM). However, in the late 1980s and early 1990s, TQM may have focused too much on one thing—quality—rather than on the entire organization. In contrast, the MBNQA was designed to focus on the entire organization, not just the one area of quality.

The initial categories were manufacturing and service, small and large. In 1999, healthcare and education were added as well.

Business results

When the winners of all of the awards are tracked over time using a hypothetical stock index, these companies have outperformed the S&P 500 Index.

One intent of the award was to provide a mechanism for sharing success stories. Winners are required to make themselves available for a period of time to tell others how they were able to achieve their results. There have been more than 30,000 presentations reaching thousands of organizations since the inception of the award. Other organizations then have the information to incorporate the learning into their businesses and create new successes.

MBNQA criteria

The MBNQA non-prescriptive criterion framework has seven categories. The business categories (manufacturing and service) are slightly different from the healthcare and education categories. The adaptations to healthcare are largely translations of the language and basic concepts of business excellence—the requirements are no less rigorous than for the other criteria. The healthcare categories include the following:

1. Leadership
2. Strategic planning
3. Focus on patients, other customers, and markets
4. Information and analysis
5. Staff focus
6. Process management
7. Organizational performance results

Categories 1 through 6 focus on key processes and category 7 focuses on results.

Each category has a maximum number of points that can be achieved. In total, there are 1,000 points available, and many organizations score about 200–300 when they begin their self-assessment. MBNQA winners usually score more than 700. The MBNQA helps direct business to achieve higher levels of performance by incorporating the sound business practices imbedded in the criteria.

Self assessment

Most businesses never get to the step of formally applying for the MBNQA. Instead, they use the criteria to conduct self-assessments and then begin to identify actions that are necessary to close the gaps. A good beginning for self-assessment is "Are We Making Progress as Leaders?" published by the National Institute of Standards and Technology. This assessment, which can be downloaded from the Baldrige National Quality Program Web site at *www.baldrige.nist.gov*, involves leadership in the review of each of the seven categories.

The table in Figure 8.1 gives some examples of the kind of questions asked of leadership.

| Figure 8.1 | Questions asked of leadership | | | | |

	Strongly disagree	Disagree	Neither agree nor disagree	Agree	Strongly agree
Category 1: Leadership Our leadership team shares information about the organization					
Category 2: Strategic planning Our employees know the parts of our organizations' plan that will affect them and their work					
Category 3: Customer and market focus Our employees ask if their customers are satisfied or dissatisfied with their work					
Category 4: Measurement, analysis, and knowledge management Our employees know how to measure the quality of their work					
Category 5: Human resource focus Our employees have a safe workplace					
Category 6: Process management Our employees can get everything they need to do their jobs					
Category 7: Business results Our employees know how well our organization is doing financially					

This is just an example of the beginning of a self-assessment process. The next step is to have leadership collectively respond to the complete tool. As they do so, they adopt the point of view of the employee on the font lines of their business.

Each year, thousands of MBNQA criteria sets are requested by organizations. Most of these organizations have found the criteria to be so powerful and in depth that they may, for the first time, recognize significant gaps in performance. The initial self-assessment alone may create actions that start to improve their businesses.

Application process

Although the self-assessment alone is valuable, applying for the award accrues additional benefits to the organization. The feedback from the examiners is generally very helpful in pointing the way to significantly improved performance.

Once the organization has decided to apply formally for the MBNQA, the first step is to obtain the current MBNQA criteria. It would be best to attend a presentation by a past winner of the MBNQA or to have one come and speak to your organization.

Then you should use an assessment and a written report to begin to understand how the criteria are applied to the organization. Organizations can conduct their own assessment or obtain training from an outside consultant to learn how to conduct one. Keep in mind that although consultants can help the organization write a refined application, they do not have the inside knowledge of how the organization works, which is required to do it in its entirety.

A team is assembled to conduct the assessment and write the application. During this time, organizations begin to identify gaps between their organization's performance and the criteria.

Once submitted to MBNQA, applications will be reviewed by examiners. If the application is considered to be excellent, a site visit is arranged for the examiners to see firsthand how well the organization is performing. The applications receive a written report addressing the areas in which there are gaps in performance to the criteria. This feedback is essential in the organization's pursuit of continuous improvement. Usually organizations go through a number of cycles of assessment and improvement before they close enough gaps to be considered for a site visit.

MBNQA examiners

Examiners are volunteers who work as a team to review MBNQA applications. Examiners have experience in applying the criteria, followed by intense training. With this new knowledge, examiners are in a better position to assist their own organizations to a new level of performance.

Healthcare organizations using Malcolm Baldrige National Quality Award

Many healthcare organizations use the MBNQA criteria as a framework based on which to improve their business. However, since the inception of the Healthcare MBNQA in 1999, only three organizations have won the award. In 2002, SSM Health Care of St. Louis, MO, won the first award, followed by Baptist Hospital, Inc., in Pensacola, FL, and Saint Luke's Hospital of Kansas City, MO, in 2003. A total of 61 applications had been submitted in the healthcare category in 2003.

Sister Mary Jean Ryan, Franciscan Sisters of Mary, president/CEO of SSM Health Care, saw how the MBNQA could improve her organization's quality and business outcomes. She and her team worked for more than seven years to get to the level of results needed to be able to win the award. As one of the largest Catholic systems in the country, the system owns, manages, and is affiliated with 21 acute care hospitals, and three nursing homes in four states (Missouri, Illinois, Wisconsin, and Oklahoma). They have about 5,000 affiliated physicians and 22,200 employees. This entire organization is assessed using the MBNQA criteria.

Similar stories of leadership were reported by Baptist Hospital and Saint Luke's Hospital. However, most MBNQA winners will tell you, **it's not about the award, but about improving business.** To do all of the work necessary just to win the award would be the wrong application of the MBNQA.

As in life generally: the reward is more in the journey than in the destination.

ISO 9000, JCAHO, and MBNQA

ISO 9000, JCAHO accreditation, and MBNQA are all standard- or criteria-based, so what is the difference between them? ISO 9000 covers about 10% of the MBNQA criteria; JCAHO covers about the same.

Because MBNQA requires demonstrable performance improvement from the seven categories, it provides a much more robust framework for businesses. Having a quality product or service but not having sound financial results is unacceptable in MBNQA. JCAHO and ISO 9000, on the other hand, do not directly address financial results.

BALDRIGE RESOURCES

"Are we making progress as Leaders?" *www.baldrige.nist.gov/Progress_Leaders.htm.*

David W. Hutton, *From Baldrige to the Bottom Line: A Road Map for Organizational Change and Improvement.*

"Getting started with the Baldrige National Quality Program," Revised March 2003, *www.baldrige.nist.gov.*

"Health Care Criteria for Performance Excellence," *www.quality.nist.gov.*

Mark Graham Brown, *Baldrige Award Winning Quality.*

Mark Graham Brown, *Keeping Score: Using the Right Metrics to Drive World-Class Performance.*

Mark Graham Brown. *Winning Score: How to Design and Implement Organizational Scorecards.*

CHAPTER NINE

RAPID CYCLE TESTING

CHAPTER NINE

RAPID CYCLE TESTING

ELEVATOR DESCRIPTION OF RAPID CYCLE TESTING

Quick: You have a two-floor ride in an elevator with your CEO and medical director and they want to know about Rapid Cycle Testing.

Rapid Cycle Testing is an expedited Plan, Do, Check, Act process. By making small improvements one at a time, a team takes on issues in bite-sized pieces and is given permission to move quickly to implement change. As with all improvement methods, it relies on a clear definition of the goal in terms of operational data.

The concepts of Rapid Cycle Testing and how they apply to healthcare can best be described in the case study that follows.

RAPID CYCLE TESTING EXAMPLE:
TIME TO CARE FOR AMBULATORY PATIENTS

An 80,000-visit-per-year emergency department (ED) had a problem with the time it took to care for ambulatory patients. As a result, patient satisfaction was low and the left-without-being-seen (LWBS) rate was high. The hospital chose to use Rapid Cycle Testing (RCT) as the improvement method for this problem.

Initial team formation. The improvement team was initially composed of the chief of emergency medicine, the assistant ED manager, a registration clerk, two triage nurses, and a staff physician working regularly in the ED.

Time allocation. The team was given one day to learn about improvement techniques (taught by a facilitator who was also a member of the group) and define the problem. It then was assigned to meet every Tuesday for three months. Each meeting was scheduled for two hours. Additional time was given to team members for implementation development and testing.

Deciding what to measure. Although reducing the LWBS rate and increasing patient satisfaction were the ultimate goals, they were not direct measures of the intake process. The team decided to measure the time from presentation to provider (physician or physician assistant) examination. At this point, a physician assistant was added to the RCT team.

Developing a measurement approach. There were a few problems with the measure they chose.

1. The ED did not collect true time of presentation. Instead, the time the patient was entered into the ED log was captured (which was sometimes after the patient waited in line for 20 minutes).

2. The team wanted to split "time to provider exam" by triage category. Unfortunately, the ED was using a new five-tier triage system, which was applied unevenly by triage nurses.

At this point, an educator was added as an ad hoc member of the team to improve the consistency of triage category assignments. In addition, a patient sign-in process was developed to better capture true time of arrival.

CASE STUDY	**RAPID CYCLE TESTING EXAMPLE: TIME TO CARE FOR AMBULATORY PATIENTS (CONT.)**

Rapid Cycle improvements

Week 1: The problem was defined and the measures established.

Week 2: A patient sign-in process was developed. Auditing was performed to capture the validity. Time of arrival was accurately entered on the sign-in sheet only 70% of the time.

Week 3: Minor changes were made to the patient sign-in process followed by brief periods of observation. The accuracy of patient presentation time was 95%. (The team continued to monitor accuracy to ensure that this was a true and sustainable change.)

Week 4: Baseline performance was measured and analyzed. Median time from presentation to provider exam was 1.5 hours for urgent, 1.7 hours for non-urgent, and 2.1 hours for minor patients. (Because "emergent" and "resuscitative" patients were seen immediately, these times were collected but not tracked.) The rate of patients LWBS was 6.5%.

Week 5: Part of the waiting process had to do with slow triage times, so the team decided to focus first on triage. The triage form was simplified and tested with staff.

Week 6: Time of triage was tracked and improved from 10 minutes to two minutes. Monitoring continued.

Week 7: A virtual fast-track system was tried. (When more than three minor or non-urgent patients were waiting, they were "treated and streeted" in one of the examination rooms.) It did not work well.

Week 8: Staffing schedules were changed, triggers were made clear, and the virtual fast-track system began to work.

Week 9: Median time from presentation to provider exam was 1.5 hours for urgent, 0.5 hours for non-urgent, and 0.6 hours for minor patients. The rate of patients leaving without being seen was 3.5%. The team now began to move its attention to urgent patients.

RAPID CYCLE TESTING CASE STUDY: TIME TO CARE FOR AMBULATORY PATIENTS (CONT.)

The team continued to meet and improve. They measured performance each week and plotted both times to provider and LWBS rates on a control chart (to distinguish "noise" from true change). It turned out that more improvements were required in the triage system and staffing changes needed to continue. However, these initial successes and the rapid nature of the changes and testing made a very big difference. The team has evolved and been replaced with new teams working on different patient-flow problems. In other words, RCT at this hospital has been a resounding success.

CHAPTER TEN

ORGANIZATIONAL ISSUES

CHAPTER TEN

ORGANIZATIONAL ISSUES

Aligning leadership

Knowing that improvement is needed and actually making improvements happen require different skills. Compare the skills necessary to enjoy golf:

- Knowing the rules of golf requires little skill, but it will enable a couch potato to enjoy an idle Sunday afternoon in front of the television set.
- Being able to have fun during 18 holes at the local golf club takes a little more skill and a lot of time at the practice tee.
- To play like a pro on the PGA tour takes talent and practice in prodigious proportions.

Being successful in quality improvement is like being successful at golf: we may know what we need to do, but to do it—and to do it well—requires specific skills. How, then, do we acquire those skills?

- Some people hire a consultant or a coach
- Some people attend conferences to learn and to meet with others with demonstrable skills
- Others, such as you, may prefer to read about the subject

Most truly successful quality professionals have benefited from all of these approaches. More importantly, they've had a chance to practice, practice, practice (just like golf!).

But no matter how skilled one becomes in quality improvement techniques, no matter how much one knows about clinical best practices or statistical process control, no matter how many "Belts" one acquires during a journey through Six Sigma, quality will not happen without the understanding, support and active participation of leadership. In fact, it is leadership that ultimately makes quality happen.

We in the quality improvement profession are at our best when we are the coaches, the facilitators, and the trainers. Executive leaders, however, are the true agents of change.

TEST YOURSELF: WHAT ARE THE ODDS?

Scenario 1: The chief of staff and chief executive officer (CEO) return from a conference where they learn that JCAHO requires demonstrable improvements in patient safety. In particular, they learn that there must be a system for the timely notification of physicians about critical test results—a system that works 100% of the time. They instruct the director of quality improvement to get a group together to assess the situation and to make improvements. They have faith that their director is the best in the business. "Just let us know what we need to do," they say as the director leaves the room. The director meets with a few people, sends out a memo of what should be done based on a thorough review of the literature, and sets about to measure and drive improvements from current performance (3σ) to optimal performance (6σ and beyond).

Question: What are the odds that there will be significant and lasting improvements?
Answer: Zero.

Scenario 2: The chief of staff and CEO return from a conference where they learn that the Joint Commission on Accreditation of Healthcare Organizations (JCAHO) requires demonstrable improvements in patient safety. In particular, they learn that there must be a system for the timely notification of physicians about critical test results—a system that works 100% of the time. They call a meeting with the director of quality improvement, the chief operating officer (COO), the chief nursing officer, the physician chair of the patient safety committee, the chief of pathology, and the chief of medicine. They ask the director of quality improvement to prepare an overview of the issue for the meeting. After a productive meeting with this small group, the chief of medicine and the COO present the issue to the administrative team, the board and the medical executive committee (MEC). The MEC and the CEO commission an improvement group, which is directed to report to these sponsors on a monthly basis until permanent improvements are realized. Performance related to this issue is placed on the board and MEC patient safety "scorecard."

Question: What are the odds that there will be significant and lasting improvements?
Answer: PDG (Pretty Darn Good).

Many quality improvement (QI) or performance improvement (PI) professionals complain that leadership is not doing what they think they should be doing. The QI professionals look at the JCAHO requirements—or other standards such as those of the Malcolm Baldrige National Quality Award or ISO 9001: 2000, and wonder how they will ever be able to document compliance.

But they may be missing the point: It is far more important to do what must be done—to do the "right thing"—than it is to show compliance with the JCAHO, ISO, or Baldrige standards. These and similar standards point us in the right direction, but lasting, meaningful, and continuous compliance only arises as a byproduct of quality. **Look past the standards and get to the real meaning of what it takes to have a "quality" organization.**

COMPLIANCE AS A BYPRODUCT OF QUALITY AND EFFICIENCY

Compliance for the sake of compliance RARELY (if ever) happens.

Compliance is only stable when it's a byproduct of quality and efficiency.

If you already believe this statement, skip this text box. If you need to be convinced, please read on.

Question: How many things do we REALLY do just because they are required?

Answer: Only those few things where enforcement is immediate and the consequences significant.

Fact: Most people drive at 70 mph on a 55 mph expressway until they see a policeman. They then slow to between 55 and 60 until they feel it safe to resume 70. Why? Because they feel 70 is a safe and effective speed.

Fact: Very few people drive 100 miles per hour regardless of the speed limit. Why? Because most people feel 100 mph is an unsafe speed. Although most people are guided by the speed limit, they will drive at what they think is a safe speed until they see a cop.

Another fact: Most people do not adhere to "stupid rules" (rules that don't seem to make sense) unless someone is looking over their shoulder.

Yet another fact: You can't look over everyone's shoulder all the time.

Conclusion: Compliance with "stupid rules" is difficult (impossible?) to maintain.

Another conclusion: To achieve compliance, eliminate all "stupid rules" by designing high quality, efficient systems that make sense and just happen to align with the JCAHO, ISO, or Baldrige standards.

Still another fact: Making "stupid rules" is easy: anyone can do it. Designing quality, efficient systems that make sense is difficult and is best done by the people who are closest to the system—at the insistence of and with the full support of executive leadership.

When executive leaders look at the resources spent on quality they often see it as "overhead" rather than an important contributor to the achievement of their strategic goals. But if an entire department is working on QI, why are the goals of leadership not included? Maybe leadership has the impression that the QI department is supposed to look only at standards outside the organization, and that the work is not supposed to be aligned with the leadership goals.

The fact is that the goals of leadership and the goals of the QI function should be mutually supportive.

Is healthcare leadership ready for change?

"Insanity is doing the same thing over and over again and expecting a different result."

—Albert Einstein

Some executive leaders freely admit they need fundamental change within their organization, but they fail to realize that to change the organization they will likely have to change the way they lead. Such fundamental change usually requires the adoption of different leadership styles inside the executive suite.

Unless leadership is ready to embrace change from within, progress will be slow, if it occurs at all. Then a new change effort is initiated, followed by another, and another, and another. This is why change initiatives often become the "flavor-of-the-month," receiving more lip service than substance: for who will invest their valuable time and reputation on a process that is likely to have but a brief shelf life. It is often easy to understand why enthusiasm and commitment for a new change effort is often hard to come by.

A 'mini' case study: One organization we know took on Total Quality Management (TQM) as its new approach to improvement. Leadership said they wanted a change, and the tools than TQM offered seemed intriguing. Other institutions were achieving remarkable results using TQM, and it seemed like a good "fit" for the organization. It quickly became apparent, however, that not everyone in the organization was fully supportive.

Why? Executive leadership adopted the trappings of TQM without understanding that, for TQM to work, they would have to change the way they managed. They continued with their familiar management styles using TQM tools and jargon as window dressing. TQM soon began to lose its luster and leadership's confidence began to wane. They ultimately moved to a new model—benchmarking and reengineering—and one of the senior leaders was heard to say, "I'm glad we don't have to do that

TQM any more, it never seemed to be an answer to our problems." Our problem, as this leader portrayed it, is that people just don't want to do what they are supposed to do. You see, the problem was the system and to other people, it had nothing to do with the folks in the executive suite.

Another senior leader said he wasn't sure the new focus on benchmarking and reengineering would work either, but he was willing to sit back and see what happened.

Did history repeat itself? Of course. When change did not come as fast as this leader wanted, blame was again assigned to the improvement method and to other people. No responsibility for the model's failure was assumed by leadership.

Why do these new improvement efforts so often fail in the healthcare industry? A large part of the problem is that leaders have been slow to appreciate that fundamental change is necessary to their core leadership style. But that's not the only reason.

Another part of the problem may be that the leaders who design and maintain institutional processes often have an interest in the status quo; they are "invested" in the current system. They are slow to give up the system they have nurtured for so long. They are also slow to take the leap of faith that the best people to design a system are those closest to it.

Another part of the problem may be the way leaders in healthcare are chosen and developed. Middle management positions, and even some offices in the executive suite, are occupied by people who are good clinicians: good nurses, skilled medical technologists, and wonderful therapists. However, those skills may not be helpful in leading a data-driven, improvement effort based in management sciences. And sometimes there just isn't a "burning platform"—that is, a crisis to serve as critical mass for such sweeping changes.

Wise leaders often enlist the aid of consultants when they recognize the need for a new improvement approach for several reasons:

- Consultants, coming from the outside, can view the organization's systems with the objective eye of someone who has not "grown up" with them.
- Consultants can be wonderful coaches: developing managers by learning from other industries and teaching the nuances of the new approach.
- And, of course, if a hospital elects to hire a consultant, it usually indicates the presence of a crisis with enough power to drive meaningful change.

Does bringing in a consultant ensure success? Certainly not. Consultants fail as often as they succeed. But in our opinion, such failures result more from the incomplete commitment of leadership than from a lack of skill on the part of the consultant.

In the final analysis, change must come from the top. It must be truly important to executive leaders or it simply will not take hold. This executive commitment seems easier to acquire in other industries, where there is one CEO and the "buck stops" at his or her desk. But healthcare is a little different. Hospital executive leaders rely on the buy-in and support of others—especially the important players of the medical staff. They are truly dependent on others when it comes to the design and management of clinical processes. This is one reason we often see change processes succeed so very well for hotel and business functions only to be derailed when they attempt to improve clinical operations.

But the fact remains: leaders who are ineffective at improving core clinical systems will be unsuccessful in driving the important improvements that will keep the institution viable. To sum it all up, change is hard in any industry. And it is much, much harder in healthcare.

How must leaders change?

- Leaders must be ready to learn new methods of leadership.
- They must create a clear, unambiguous vision of the hospital's direction.
- Leaders must be effective in communicating the vision to all employees and stakeholders, including physicians.
- They must provide the resources necessary to achieve this vision.

This clear, unambiguous vision must guide leaders' actions and the actions of their subordinates. In short, they must walk the walk.

These responsibilities cannot be delegated to other levels in the organization. Executive leaders themselves must demonstrate the change they are calling upon others to make. They must reinforce their vision, based on a viable strategic plan, every day—in the way they hold subordinates accountable, in the way they recognize achievement . . . in the way they manage.

But this is why Six Sigma, Lean Thinking, Rapid Cycle Testing, and other quality methodologies are able to deliver results. They set out a structure for leading, based on data and scientific management methods. The tools are more than window dressing, and the improvement method is more than an aspect of the organization: the tools and the methods ARE the way leaders lead.

HOW LEADERS LEAD

What are some of the characteristics of leaders who are ready for change? They

- make the work a priority and are persistent.
- provide direction—and a clear definition of the objectives.
- provide resources to get the work done.
- make time for updates to staff.
- provide recognition and rewards for achievements.
- provide support for the work being done.
- assign the best people possible to the work.
- remove barriers if no one else is able to.
- involve everyone associated with the work—there are no favorites or exclusions.
- don't quit when the journey gets tough.

Is leadership ready to write the check/make resources available?

When leadership contemplates whether to provide a new service, the costs and benefits of the change must be evaluated. After careful review of the data, leadership decides whether or not to invest in the new service.

The process for deciding on the adoption of a new quality approach is exactly the same. The approach must make sense, support the business plan and goals of the organization, and create a return on the investment. If these criteria are demonstrable to leadership, it's time to write the check. But how big is that check?

Funding a robust improvement program does not necessarily mean building a larger quality department. However, it usually means that someone from the quality department must be available to help leaders with implementation and to facilitate improvement teams.

Ideally, managers become trained to support their own improvement efforts with additional support from other departments involved in the process and the quality department supporting the ongoing training and team facilitation. Ultimately, resources for improvement are funded out of departmental budgets.

Prioritizing projects

Improvement starts with focus. Leaders must identify their key business processes and markets. They must define their primary operational objectives. These considerations allow the selection of key improvement projects—those that will significantly improve the organization's performance and bottom line. The best candidates for improvement are business lines that are losing money or market share and those that are easiest to measure.

JCAHO standard LD.4.50 outlines how to prioritize the performance improvement efforts. Over the years quality departments have developed complex matrices to demonstrate the prioritization process for surveyors. But we counsel simplicity: simply list the strategic goals of the organization and show alignments between those goals and improvement projects underway.

It is customary and productive to conduct a SWOT analysis to assist the prioritization of potential projects.

SWOT ANALYSIS

The analysis begins with the business plan, which describes the key business goals of the organization. Each phase of the business plan is assessed for the following four elements:

S = strengths (Where is the business particularly strong?)

W = weaknesses (Which phases of the business need significant improvement?)

O = opportunities (Are there opportunities at hand for business enhancements?)

T = threats (Which aspects of the business are currently under attack?)

A business plan should describe current market strengths, organization strengths and weaknesses, competitors, opportunities for improvement, and external threats to the current or projected market share. Doing such a SWOT analysis will generate a list of goals and, perhaps, strategies for improvement. These goals, or priorities, serve as the basis for team-driven improvements that are run though your improvement method of choice.

We discussed the strategic planning cycle in the section on Balanced Scorecards in Chapter 6. This section will describe how one hospital uses the strategic planning cycle to drive improvements, using traditional TQM approaches and a balanced scorecard.

Defining 'strategic'

Let's take another look a the strategic planning cycle, illustrated in Figure 10.1.

Figure 10.1	**Strategic planning cycle**

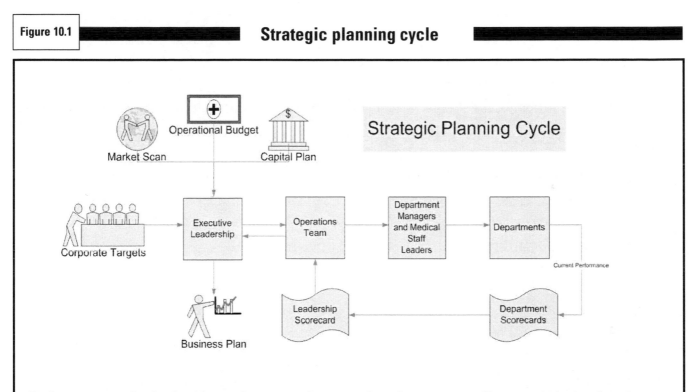

Each year, executive leadership receives strategic targets from the corporate office, scans the local market and develops operational and capital budgets. This is summarized in an updated business plan. Departmental and leadership scorecards that are aligned with this business plan are then measured on an ongoing basis.

The first part of the cycle involves developing the business plan and, correspondingly, the strategic goals.

What is going to make your organization stay at the top of the market? What needs to be done to continue to stay in business and to provide the services needed in the community? Most solid organizations undergo ongoing planning to develop strategic goals aimed at keeping the hospital solvent and moving forward. A strategic goal is different from a financial goal in that

- financial goals are fundamental to business; they are necessary to keep a for-profit corporation solvent and to give a not-for-profit organization the ability to borrow funds. Without meeting financial targets, it ultimately becomes difficult to pay the bills, to hire the staff, and to stay in business.

- strategic goals are features of the operations that allow the institution to reach its financial goals.

"But wait," you say. "A hospital is more than a business, its part of a community infrastructure. In some cases, it's the fulfillment of a higher social mission."

True. But if the hospital cannot achieve its financial goals, its ability to achieve its higher, social function is diminished.

On the other hand, some CEOs and some hospital chains seem to focus only on finances without appreciating the strategic and community benefit layers of a healthcare institution (see Figure 10.2). Although the finances-only approach often succeeds in the short term, it usually diminishes the long-term viability of the institution.

| Figure 10.2 | **Strategic and community benefit layers** |

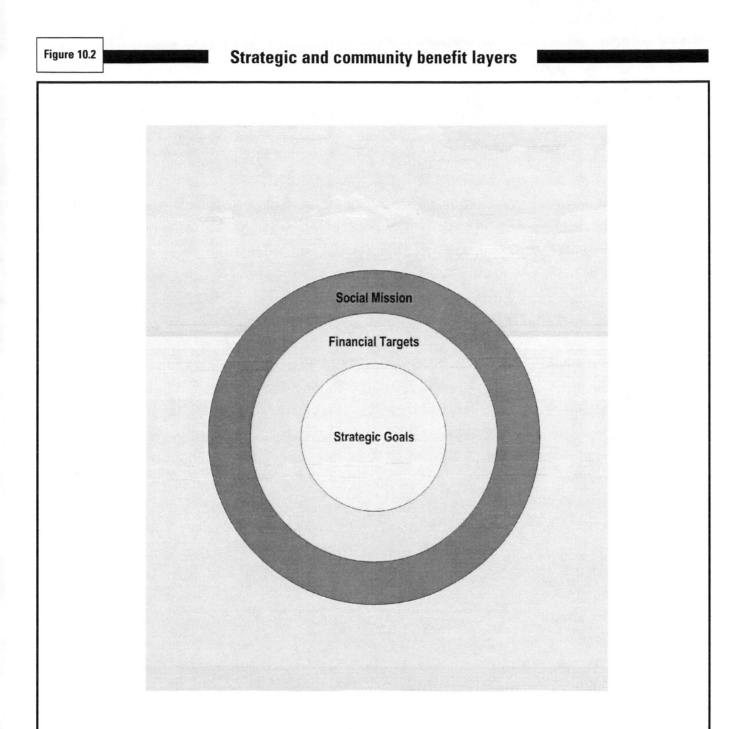

Strategic goals pertain to the operational processes that will help an organization attain financial goals in concert with the external environment.

Jack Welch, the well-publicized CEO of General Electric (GE), knew the financial picture of his organization intimately. But finances were not his focus. He focused on reducing defects using Six Sigma.

You see, he realized that satisfied customers drove sales, which drove finances. Defective products do not make customers happy. He also recognized the link between defects and higher production costs due to defects.

He could have focused on cost-cutting measures to meet the budget. He could have told people that the budget wasn't being met. He could have implored his employees to "get better" at what they were doing. He could have fired those employees not meeting their budgets. He could have chosen to do many things, but none of them would have addressed the root cause of GE's problems.

Instead, Welch became very successful by creating better systems.

Good healthcare leaders, like successful captains of industry, need to focus staff on more than finances. They must focus the organization on the operational and community processes that lead to institutional health. But this focus must be specific; leaders must set objective, measurable targets.

When hospitals set strategic goals with measurable targets, they commonly sort the goals into the following categories:

- Finance
- Service
- Clinical quality
- Human resources
- Community

We will discuss these categories—this framework for a set of strategic goals—as we go.

Deploying the business plan

This collection of strategic goals and targets is the business plan, but the plan won't do much good unless it's deployed.

What about secrets in business plan? What about nuggets of information that could pose a threat to the organization if they were known by competitors or contractors? Such considerations are why some institutions never let the business plan out of the CEO's office. But there is no reason the thrust of the business plan cannot or should not be used to align priorities for improvement. Why not just transform the thrust of the business plan into a list of strategic goals and targets? This approach strikes the right balance in many institutions.

Setting overall targets and specific department measures

The next step in the process is developing clear targets in each area of the business plan and creating a method for encouraging improvement (and holding managers accountable for more than just finances). Refer to Chapter 6 and Figure 6.4 to see what an organization's effort looks like with many good people working as hard as they can in the direction that they individually think is most important. This kind of process lacks clear direction from leadership. Refer to Figure 6.5 to see what an organization's effort looks like with many good people working as hard as they can in a direction set by leadership.

Finance

No one would start a year without a budget. Managers are used to being measured in terms of variance to budget. This will not change. What should change, however, is that managers also be held accountable for goals in the other domains (such as clinical quality, service, human resources and community service).

Service

Knowing what customers or patients think about an organization is extremely important to the business. When customers' needs are not meet, they usually vote with their feet and take their business someplace else. Therefore, patient satisfaction is commonly measured and can serve as an overall goal for the institution. However, like a departmental budget, each functional area would be held accountable for satisfaction within their service area.

What about support departments, functions that do not provide direct services? Some institutions have chosen to hold these departments accountable for overall patient satisfaction and customer satisfaction.

Clinical quality

Clinical quality should be the hallmark of any healthcare organization. It is the foundation of the organization's reputation, important to staff and physicians, and the best form of risk management. However, clinical quality in the abstract should be focused by the specific services given by the institution. For example, if your organization has a regional heart program, then those measures of performance should be on your strategic goal list. If you want to increase the market in OB care, then those measures should be on your strategic goal list.

- Some departments select targets for fundamental care issues—for example, pain management, medication processes, or National Patient Safety Goals.
- Some departments set targets for care to given patient populations, such as time to intervention for patients with acute myocardial infarction, time to antibiotic therapy for pneumonia patients, risk-adjusted perinatal morbidity and mortality, etc.
- Some support departments select targets for important services to clinical departments, such as STAT room cleaning times for environmental services.

Human resources

Key human resources functions include recruitment, retention, and training. It is important that each department receive reports and be held accountable for indicators related to these functions, such as

- retention or turnover rates (new and existing employees)
- employee commitment (satisfaction)
- completion of employee training

Community—Corporate citizen

It is important to be in tune with the community's needs. The organization should determine how it can partner with the community. For example,

- if the community is aging, then it would be important to provide flu and pneumovac shots at no or low cost.
- if the community is younger and in an area that has a large amount of swimming pools, then a community outreach on pool safety would be ideal.
- if the community has a lot of children who ride bikes, a community service might include bike safety, such as the need to wear bike helmets.
- if the community has a population of young teenage girls becoming pregnant, then a do-not-abandon-your-baby campaign may be appropriate.

Strategic goals with target numbers

Once leadership has decided which goals are most important, they then must decide how to measure them. Goals that are measurable have a chance of being actionable. But how often should a goal be measured? As often as you want a chance to work on the issue. If an issue is important, it is best to measure at least monthly. If it is a process that has rapid turnaround, then weekly or daily works well. To see whether action plans are working, it is better to have feedback more frequently.

Unless something changes, it is hard to remember what intervention worked well, especially if there are multiple action steps. Therefore, measures should be collected as close to the process as possible and then reported on quickly. You may waste time if you wait months to measure, especially if what you measured doesn't provide the improvement you sought.

Some goals are not numeric

Sometimes a goal doesn't lend itself to a numeric endpoint. For example, the goal may be to implement a plan. In such a case, measure milestones toward the goal). Make an implementation plan with specific targets along the way.

Who should determine the goals?

Who should determine the overall goals of the organization? Senior leaders and possibly the board of directors, but, there should be buy-in from the principal owners of the process or principal uses of the process. Physician groups that use the services also should be consulted to get their input on what the organization is trying to achieve and the goals it is targeting. And don't forget the middle managers!

Rolling goals though the organization

A worksheet should be developed to help guide managers as they develop goals and targets for their individual departments. These are collected and approved by leadership and then managers are rewarded and otherwise held accountable for the entire scope of performance . . . not just finances. Figure 10.3 is a blank sample of a strategic goals worksheet for you to keep deployment of a plan on track. Figure 10.4 is a sample of a completed strategic goals worksheet. To keep track of your goals in a scorecard (refer to Chapter 6 for more on scorecards and another example in figure 6.6), refer to Figure 10.5

Figure 10.3 **Blank strategic goals worksheet**

Goal Area	Strategic Goals	Actions or Strategies
Finance	Specific Strategic Goals	Specific Actions or Strategies
Service	Specific Strategic Goals	Specific Actions or Strategies
Clinical Quality	Specific Strategic Goals	Specific Actions or Strategies
Human Resources	Specific Strategic Goals	Specific Actions or Strategies
Community –Corporate Citizen	Specific Strategic Goals	Specific Actions or Strategies

> **Figure 10.4** ▬▬▬▬ **Sample completed strategic goals worksheet** ▬▬▬▬

Area	Strategic goals	Actions or strategies
Finance	• OB hospital days will be X • The monthly budget will be within X% of goal	• Monitor payroll and nonpayroll costs • Monitor overtimes and incidental costs
Service	• Increase OB satisfaction scores to X% • Review Federal Emergency Medical Treatment and Active Labor Act (EMTALA)	• Improve pain management during labor • Improve information given to new mothers regarding self care and baby care • Improve the discharge process • Review processes to support appropriate EMTALA requirements
Clinical quality	• Improve pain management during labor • Improve information given to new mothers regarding self care and baby care • Conduct preoperative or invasive procedure briefings	• Pain assessment skills for nurses • Pain management with anesthesia • Develop new mother and baby educational process
Human Resources	• Reduce turnover rate for first- year nurses • Reduce turnover rate for nurses employed more than one year • Reduce vacancy rate	• Assess needs of new nurses • Preceptor program for new nurses • Employ patient safety briefings to improve teamwork • Assess needs of nurses employed more than one year • Hire the best nurses available and retain them
Community – Corporate Citizen	• Reduce incidence in the community of abandoned babies	• Develop campaign to work with at-risk groups regarding a "Do Not Abandon Your Baby" program

Figure 10.5 ▮▮▮▮▮ Strategic goals scorecard ▮▮▮▮▮

(ORGANIZATION NAME) (DEPARTMENT NAME) (DATE) STRATEGIC GOALS SCORECARD *(Mission Statement)*			

Affordability *Affordable Care*	☺	😐	☹	**Clinical Quality** *Quality You Can Trust*	☺	😐	☹
• OB hospital days will XX.				• Improve pain management during labor.			
• The monthly budget will be within XX% of goal				• Improve information given to the new mother regarding self care and for baby care			
• Monitor payroll and non payroll costs				•			
Monitor overtimes costs • Monitor incidental costs				•			
Personalized Care				•			
Access - *Convenient and Easy Access*				•			
• EMTALA Review				•			
Perception of Services - *Caring with a Personal Touch*							
• Increase our OB Satisfaction Scores to XX%				**Regulatory Compliance**			
• Improve the discharge process to reduce wait time for transportation to less than XX				• Effective Continuous Compliance Program			
Safety Experience				**People & Systems** *People Being Supported by Effective Systems*			
• Conduct pre- pre-operative or invasive procedure briefings				• Reduce turn over rate for first year nurses to less than 1%			
•				• Reduce turnover rate for nurses employed more than one year to less than 1%			
•				• Reduce vacancy rate for RN staff to less than 1%			
				Community Service			
				• Address community needs with Baldwin Park Community Benefits *(Plan)*	☺		

Note
This scorecard is based on results received as of ------, 200X.
Performance is reflected to the right of the goal.
The target is reflected in the parenthesis *(in italic)* next to the goal.

KEY
↑ = significant improvement over past performance
☺ = exceeding, meeting or –1% from accomplishing the target
😐 = close but not quite there (greater than 1% away from accomplishing target but not exceeding 5% away from target)
☹ = needs more work (greater than 5% away from accomplishing the target)

Goals should be communicated to the organization

There are many ways to communicate your goals. Tools of communication that your organization may already be using or could easily and inexpensively create include the following:

- Newsletters
- Payday mailers
- Leaders visiting departments in person
- Incentive pay, if possible

How often should goals be measured or updated?

How often should data be collected and displayed? The answer is really how often you want a chance to evaluate how well action plans are working. How often do you want a chance to make a difference? It is recommended that the measures be updated and shared with staff monthly, but it depends on your organization. Some measures are available only on a quarterly basis. As a general rule, update goals when new data are available.

A hospital is located in a "bedroom community" on the outskirts of a large urban area. Long-term economic projections for the region are rosy and the relatively young, married customer base led leadership to put the enhancement of reproductive services high on its strategic plan. Their vision: to become the reproductive "provider of choice" for the community.

Are the hospital's existing reproductive services in a good position to meet this growing demand and achieve this lofty vision? Let's look at its high-level SWOT analysis.

Strengths:

- The hospital is affiliated with the leading obstetrical group in the community and works with a growing number of smaller obstetrical practices.

- The inpatient perinatal service (labor, delivery, postpartum, normal newborn) had a good reputation and was able to recruit and retain a strong staff of nurses.

Weaknesses:

- Patient satisfaction with the labor and delivery service is in the 45th percentile of all similar services polled by the hospital's satisfaction contractor. The hospital found two issues at the root of this dissatisfaction: management of pain and the physical environment.

- The labor and delivery unit was built in 1984 and would need to be redesigned and expanded to meet the aggressive growth projected for the community.

- The hospital does not have a high-acuity special care nursery. A nearby community hospital has a level III intensive care nursery and a good reputation. Most high-risk antepartum patients are therefore admitted to their competitor.

<table>
<tr><td>**CASE STUDY**</td><td>**USING A STRATEGIC GOAL TO PRIORITIZE IMPROVEMENT PROJECTS (CONT.)**</td></tr>
</table>

Opportunities:

- The community's leading obstetrical group is interested in developing an in vitro fertilization clinic in cooperation with the community.

Threats:

- A nearby competitor is seeking financing for the creation of a low-risk, modern "birthing center."

What part can TQM, Six Sigma, Lean Thinking, Benchmarking, or other quality improvement processes play in realizing leadership's vision? Is there an improvement project that can advance the perinatal service?

You may have come up with other options, but we feel that the best bet is working on pain management as it relates to patient satisfaction.

APPENDIX ONE

OVERREACTING TO CHANGE

OVERREACTING TO CHANGE

How often do we report numbers quarterly/annually or without context and hope to make sense of them?

✓ "In 2003 our delinquency rate was 34%. This year, 2004, it was 42%. There must be something wrong!"

✓ "Our performance went up last month. Let's have a pizza party!"

Are these appropriate reactions, or are these examples of damaging "tampering" or overreaction?

Figure A.1   **Two points**

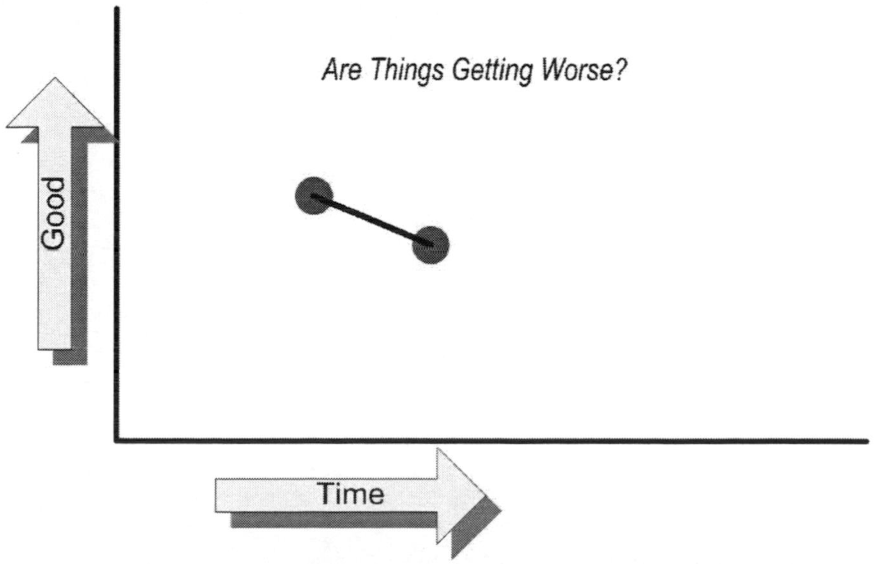

Are Things Getting Worse?

Good

Time

Results diminish from one reporting period to the next. Are things getting worse? It depends on context.

We've spent a lot of time talking about the importance of holding people accountable for performance and celebrating success, but reacting based on only two data points may not be the right way to do it. In fact, Shewhart and others have described the damage leaders can cause by tampering with systems in response to routine variation.

The only way to know if the difference between two numbers represents a change is to put those two numbers in context:

1. Always report numbers with as much historical performance as possible.
2. Report data points with sufficient frequency to allow leaders to review change in context.

Figure A.2 Data in context

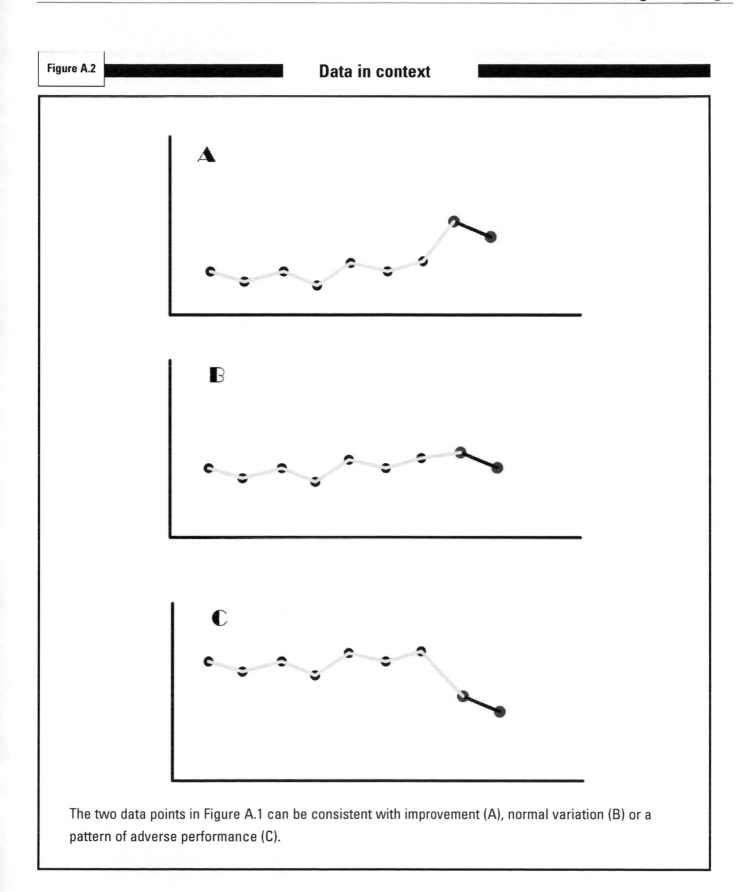

The two data points in Figure A.1 can be consistent with improvement (A), normal variation (B) or a pattern of adverse performance (C).

APPENDIX TWO

STORYBOARDS FOR RECOGNITION AND COMMUNICATION

STORYBOARDS FOR RECOGNITION AND COMMUNICATION

One hospital we know started displaying storyboards during a JCAHO survey many years ago. The hospital got a perfect score (grid score of 100), which provided good reinforcement for the storyboard process (even though it was not clear how much the storyboards contributed to survey success). Did the storyboards impress JCAHO? Yes. But, more importantly, it impressed hospital staff and leadership. It communicated the story of success and boosted ongoing improvement efforts.

Using simple storyboards is an excellent way to communicate improvement results throughout the organization. Some hospitals have routine storyboard competitions, with a recognition luncheon for all involved. Storyboards are condensed displays of a system's performance over time. Although storyboards can be elaborate undertakings costing many hundreds of dollars in graphics (the kind you often see at conferences) we prefer simple, modest efforts that tell the story of success in a glance. When we talk about a storyboard we think of a single 8 $\frac{1}{2}$ x 11 inch piece of paper, with domains representing each step in your improvement process.

In the following example, we assume that the improvement process is "Plan, Measure, Assess, Improve." However, you may wish to use "Plan, Do, Study, Act" or "Design, Measure, Assess, Improve, Control," or whatever model you prefer.

Here's what we put in each of the domains on our storyboards:

Domain 1: Plan

> **a. Problem identification:** Look for changes in important business indicators. Use strategic goals, supporting proxy measures for the strategic goals, and important operational measures that reveal gaps in performance.

Tools: Brainstorming; scorecards; other data confirming problem

    b. Mission/Goal: What should performance look like when you are done? Use a numeric goal when possible.

    Tools: Brainstorming; timelines

Domain 2: Measure. Display data about a performance/results of a process. Describe patterns or trends in a process and assist in identifying root causes.

    Tools: Data collection; control/run charts (statistical process control); histograms; cause and effect diagrams; Pareto charts; flowcharts

Domain 3: Assess. Analyze data to develop information about a process and identify the root cause(s). Confirm opinions on root cause(s) with data whenever possible.

    Tools: Root cause analysis; ask the five whys: who, what, where, when, and with whom?; cause and effect diagram; Pareto charts; flowcharts

Domain 4: Improve.

    a. Actions: Describe actions taken to change a process based on organizational priorities and control measures instituted.

    Tools: Gantt charts; decision matrices; control charts

    b. Measure: Display the results of your improvements in terms of improved process data.

    Tools: Control charts, Pareto diagrams

RELATED PRODUCTS

The Greeley Company
200 Hoods Lane, Marblehead, MA 01945
TEL: 888/749-3054   **E-MAIL:** *tgc@greeley.com*   **FAX:** 781/639-0085
WEB: *www.greeley.com*

The Greeley Company—a national leader in educational and consulting services for hospitals and other healthcare organizations—offers a wide range of accreditation and patient safety services tailored to your organization's specific needs.

Our award-winning team of experts offers both consulting and onsite education modules to train physicians and medical staff professionals, survey coordinators, quality staff, administrators, compliance officers/personnel, liability/risk-reduction professionals, and other healthcare professionals. We provide expert guidance and detailed systems/process reviews, policies and procedures development, and interim staffing.

Our focus areas include:

Patient Safety and Quality

- **Patient Safety and Medical Error Reduction:** Through The Greeley Company's partnership with Performance Improvement International, you will get practical strategies to reduce medical errors, conduct effective RCAs and FMEAs, analyze sentinel events, and comply with JCAHO standards.

- **Quality and Performance Improvement:** Receive measurable worthwhile improvements to patient care, clinical outcomes, and workflow efficiencies, while enhancing cost savings.

- **Making Peer Review Effective:** Improve your physician peer review process to make it more fair, confidential, positive, and effective. Our experts will help you with both assessments and implementation.

Accreditation

- **JCAHO Organizational Self-Assessment Services:** Correctly complete JCAHO's new self-assessment by having our experts review applicable standards, relevant dimensions of performance, and systems and processes.

- **JCAHO Survey Preparation:** Our survey experts provide practical, engaging survey preparation, in compliance with JCAHO's new tracer methodology survey process and to prepare for the upcoming random unannounced surveys in 2006

- **Accreditation Interim Staffing:** The Greeley Company's interim staffing professionals can help you to overcome your temporary staffing needs and help prepare you for a successful JCAHO survey.

Clinical Operations Improvement

- **Coping with Hospital and E.D. Overcrowding Crisis:** Hospitals are spending millions of capital dollars to expand their emergency departments only to find that new beds fill quickly and patients continue to languish in the emergency department for lack of appropriate placement. The Greeley Company, in collaboration with InSight Advantage, can help you quickly turn this trend around through our comprehensive, practical, and cost-effective process for optimizing patient flow.

- **Boosting Finances by Improving Patient Flow**
  The Greeley Company will provide concrete steps to improve your facility's patient flow to augment organizational finances and comply with the JCAHO's new patient flow standard LD.3.11 (effective January 1, 2005). Through our three-step process, we will assess your patient-flow process— from intake at the emergency department to inpatient discharge—develop scorecards to identify bottlenecks and track improvements, and present practical strategies for improvement.

The Greeley Company also offers extensive consulting and educational services in credentialing and privileging, medical staff office assessment and interim staffing, core privileging, board education and leadership development, liability risk reduction, department and service-line assessments, medical staff leadership development, medical staff bylaws, external peer review, legal support, and much more.

To learn more about The Greeley Company's onsite education programs or consulting services, please call us toll-free at 888/749-3054, or e-mail us at *tgc@greeley.com* Your initial consultation is free.